IMAGES
of America

EVANSTON HOSPITAL
SCHOOL OF NURSING
1898–1984

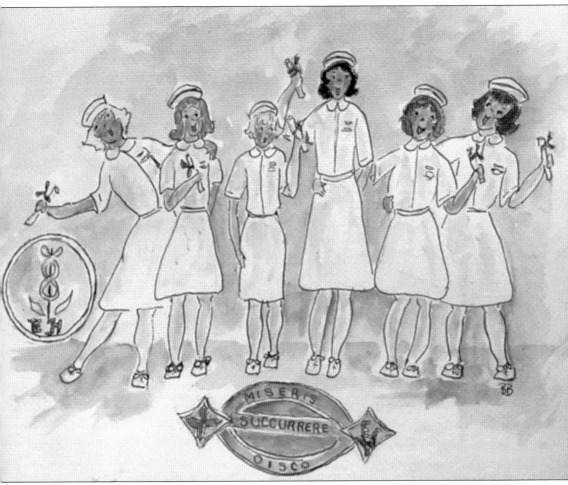

Nationally renowned artist Bonnie Bowen captured all the emotions of becoming a nurse on graduation day—joy, happiness, and pride—in her painting *A Look Back*. She created the whimsical watercolor painting as a gift to the 1972 Evanston Hospital School of Nursing (EHSN) graduates in celebration of their 50th anniversary reunion. From 1901 to 1984, EHSN graduates displayed the same emotions when receiving their diploma and pin. (Bonnie Bowen.)

ON THE COVER: EHSN students are pictured in the science laboratory of Patten Memorial Hall, which was built in 1930. James and Amanda Patten made financial contributions for the construction of this building, as they did in 1910 for the first nursing residence, Patten Hall, in memory of James's brother George. (Archives of NorthShore University HealthSystem.)

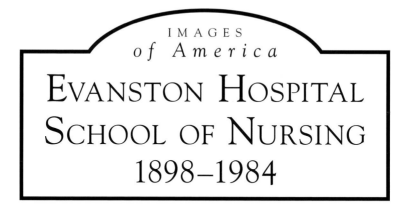

IMAGES
of America

EVANSTON HOSPITAL
SCHOOL OF NURSING
1898–1984

Carolyn Hope Smeltzer
and Barbara Ann McQuillan
Foreword by John Tressa

ARCADIA
PUBLISHING

Published by Arcadia Publishing
Charleston, South Carolina

Printed in the United States of America

Library of Congress Control Number: 2022937400

For all general information, please contact Arcadia Publishing:
Telephone 843-853-2070
Fax 843-853-0044
E-mail sales@arcadiapublishing.com
For customer service and orders:
Toll-Free 1-888-313-2665

Visit us on the Internet at www.arcadiapublishing.com

To the memory of Marjorie Beyers (1936–2022): a strong and thoughtful leader, a conceptual thinker, a humble person, and simply brilliant. She was a mentor and supporter to many. She impacted nurses' lives without forgetting her roots growing up on a farm. She was a gentle soul with a continuous smile.

To all Evanston Hospital School of Nursing graduates, especially the class of 1972, and the faculty members who created a heritage of caring and left a legacy of the art, science, and heart of providing excellent care to patients.

CONTENTS

FOREWORD

As I walk through the employee entrance corridor at Evanston Hospital each day, I take time to browse the photographs of the hospital's rich history and am always especially inspired by the photographs of the Evanston Hospital School of Nursing and all of the students who received their nursing education there. It is incredible to imagine the stories and contributions of the student nurses and nursing educators who provided the inspiration, guidance, and strong diploma nursing education over the school's 86-year history.

When Carolyn and I first spoke of this book and her incredible labor of love to create it, so many vivid and wonderful memories were triggered of my own diploma nursing education at Ravenswood Hospital Medical Center School of Nursing in the early 1980s. Having been exposed to nursing for all of my life through my mom, a 42-year nurse and hospital school of nursing diploma graduate, it seemed inevitable that I would follow the same path. As I began my journey to decide where I would receive my nursing education, my mom was quite insistent that I choose a university setting and a bachelor of science in nursing as my entry into nursing practice. While I applied and was accepted to several phenomenal BSN programs, my heart and head always brought me back to the diploma program that I was also accepted to. The feel, the warmth, and the commitment to day-one nursing education and clinical experience let me know that I made the right choice. While nursing education has forever changed, those days in my diploma program made me the nurse that I am today and so grateful to be.

Thank you, Carolyn and Barbara, for telling the stories of the Evanston Hospital School of Nursing, and for sharing your experiences and those of your classmates at this remarkable school. Your stories give hope and inspiration to so many of us who share the diploma nursing education experience, as well as those who wish to learn and share our treasured memories for years to come.

—John Tressa, DNP (Candidate), MSN, MBA, RN, NE-BC
Chief Nursing Officer, NorthShore University HealthSystem

ACKNOWLEDGMENTS

The authors would first like to thank Evanston Hospital School of Nursing and its faculty for giving students a value-driven educational experience with opportunities to provide nursing care to diverse patients with complex needs. Without excellent and committed faculty from the beginning in 1898, there would have been no school to write about.

This book would not have been possible without several leaders of NorthShore University HealthSystem who understood the value of and need to preserve the history of EHSN. We want to extend a special thank-you to Nancy Semerdjian, retired chief nurse officer of NorthShore University HealthSystem, who worked with and respected so many EHSN graduates throughout her tenure. Without hesitancy, Semerdjian described the purpose and value of the proposed book to J.P. Gallagher, the president and chief executive officer of NorthShore University HealthSystem. Gallagher was very supportive of the project and identified individuals who had access to the school's vintage photographs. Thanks also to Jim Anthony, senior director of public relations; Linda Feinberg, director of NorthShore Library Services; and Maggie Panicker, training coordinator of nursing professional development and research, all of whom were instrumental in graciously retrieving the historic images used in this book. They believed the history of the school should not just be in archival files but in a publication that can be shared by all. Unless otherwise noted, all images in this book are from the archives of NorthShore University HealthSystem.

Thanks to the family of Marjorie Beyers who understood her important role in nursing and remembered her talking fondly about her time at EHSN. Marjorie's family shared memories, articles, letters, booklets, and pictures that she had cherished and saved.

Many 1972 graduates of EHSN provided memories, stories, notes, and photographs for this book: Susan Iris (Bermann) Keener, Mary Gerarda (Callahan) Blaisdell, Roseann Elizabeth (Ciaccio) Boi, Cheryl (Duba) Petersen, Roberta Joanne Hilliger, Rebecca Jane Jelinek-Simon, Janelle/Janice Elaine (Kronbold) Adamski, Karen (Jones) Waechter, Linda Sue "Lenny" (Lenart) Cranford, Barbara (Paul) Schroeder, Carol Ann (Rumney) Beebe, Nancy June (Schupp) Miller, Sandra (Green) Sill, Frances Marie (Vretis) Skafidas, and Katherine Ann (Willy) Carroll. These graduates, along with Kathryn (Horton) Gray, made the school's history come alive.

Thanks to Jeff Ruetsche, acquisitions editor, and Caroline Anderson Vickerson, title manager, from Arcadia Publishing for believing the history, stories, vintage images, and memories of EHSN would be of interest to many and an illustrative example of diploma nursing schools during the time when EHSN was in operation. They recognized that this book would demonstrate nursing diploma educational values and historical relevance. Jeff and Caroline were aware of the aging population of diploma nursing graduates and agreed that now was the perfect time to record their history. Both challenged the authors to find clear, crisp, and interesting images coupled with relevant captions to make the book engaging, meaningful, and lasting.

INTRODUCTION

The Evanston Hospital School of Nursing class of 1972 selected three songs for their graduation ceremony, which was held on June 17: "A Time for Us" by Nina Rota, "Morning has Broken" by Cat Stevens, and "The Impossible Dream" by Leigh and Darion. These songs were sung by the class soloist, Linda DuBien.

"A Time for Us" was the theme song from the 1969 movie *Romeo and Juliet*, which was released in theaters the same year these students entered EHSN. During freshman year, the nursing class voted "A Time for Us" to be their theme song. When a student got engaged, pinned, or married, a buzzer would ring in each dormitory room to signify that a fellow student had a special occasion. The buzzer usually rang when the students were sleeping or studying in their pajamas. Each student would hurry to the auditorium in Patten Memorial Hall to find out who they would be celebrating. The special student would be placed in the middle of a circle with the other students around her, holding hands, and singing "A Time for Us." This ritual occurred for the next three years.

"Morning has Broken" was first published in 1931. The Cat Stevens version of this peaceful hymn became popular in 1971. The 1972 class president and resident hippie, Roberta Hilliger, continuously played the song in her dormitory room in Patten Memorial Hall. She used it to relax and meditate when she was stressed from providing patient care, studying for class, or just living life. Every Friday night, after classes ended, Hilliger would play Cat Stevens, wait for her girlfriend to get off work, and then go out for an Italian dinner.

"The Impossible Dream" is from the 1965 Broadway musical *Man of La Mancha*. Ironically, this was the same year many of the class of 1972 decided on nursing as their career. This song was recommended by DuBien, who had a beautiful voice that many of her classmates still remember 50 years later. She lived in the dormitory for only one year; she got married and had a baby before starting her senior year. DuBien used public transportation to travel to and from school, many times with her baby, making her graduation seem almost like an impossible dream.

Each chapter in this book is named after a line from one of the songs performed by DuBien at the 1972 pinning and graduation ceremony. The reader will soon recognize this book is not solely about EHSN. The history and students' experiences described and the images displayed throughout are merely a platform to illustrate the history of diploma nursing schools.

The first chapter provides a description of how the sick were originally cared for, the evolution of Evanston Hospital, and the need for trained nurses in the United States. Evanston Hospital and its nursing school serve as an example of the evolution of the country's health care system. This chapter describes why it was "a time for us" to start training professional nurses to provide care in hospitals rather than continuing the practice of having women of religious orders or inexperienced women provide nursing care in homes.

This chapter also explains the connectivity of Evanston Emergency Hospital and the training school that became EHSN. Hospitals around the country needed staff trained to provide care, which led to the growth of diploma nursing programs. As at other hospitals, Evanston Emergency Hospital's leadership recognized a need to have trained nursing staff. The hospital developed a nursing school seven years after Evanston Emergency Hospital was founded in 1891. In the early years of the Evanston Training School for Nurses, upon entering the school, students were not charged tuition for their education, and when they finished the program, the nurse graduates were awarded $100 for their service.

The book's second chapter gives the reader a burst of insight into the first 50 years at EHSN. Through images of students, the dormitory, and the classrooms, readers can get a feel for what it was like to attend nursing school between the years of 1898 and 1948. When the school first opened, the students had at least 72-hour work weeks, which included clinical studies, lectures, and study time. The school's curriculum, the students' studies, and their types of work in the hospital are explored. Although this chapter highlights EHSN's history with vintage photographs from that specific school, it also demonstrates the life of many nursing students attending any diploma school during this period.

This chapter may have the reader wanting to inquire into their own nursing school's history, perhaps wondering how and why their own school of nursing was started, who the leaders were, and what it was like being trained during this era. The EHSN students who were trained over 125 years ago had unimaginable hours to keep as well as strict rules to follow. On their second day after entering the school, the students reported to hospital wards to care for patients. The Evanston Training School for Nurses students had 12-hour days or nights providing patient care. Their classes generally started at 8:00 in the evening, and sometimes—but not always—the students would be granted a half day off for free time on Sundays. When a student nurse wanted to leave the hospital premises, she needed permission from the nursing superintendent. Readers of this chapter may gain an appreciation for those student nurses and faculty who paved the way for future student nurses to have a more effective educational process along with less restrictive living conditions.

The third chapter narrates how EHSN positioned itself to be an attractive choice for high school students who wanted to be nurses. By 1960, a large portion of Illinois hospitals had their own educational programs for nursing students. Many hospitals were sponsored by a religious group or had an ethnic origin, which gave them an edge in describing their school's mission. Nursing schools had to be proactive and competitive to attract students. EHSN faculty created a booklet positioning the school as a special place that could offer any student an outstanding experience. This booklet, developed in the 1960s, advertised why EHSN was "a place for us" and encouraged potential students to choose EHSN after selecting nursing as their future profession. This chapter highlights the curriculum, outstanding faculty, cost of attending EHSN, and dormitory life. The booklet proudly described EHSN offering each student a private single room in a dormitory with an elegant reception lounge where students could gather and socialize. It outlines the requirements to be accepted as a student as well as the opportunities for work after graduation; it also references the school's ability to prepare students to be good wives and mothers.

While reading chapter three, readers may dig into their own memories to recognize why they chose nursing as a career and how they decided which nursing school to attend. When Linda Cranford, a 1972 EHSN graduate, was asked these questions, she replied, "It's a funny story, I was going to be a secretary. In my senior year I worked with a nurse in sick bay. She invited me to come along with a group to visit EHSN. Once there, I fell in love with it. With Lake Michigan just blocks away and what I thought was an enchanting school, I was sure this was where I wanted to be. Of the 10 high school seniors, I was the only one that chose an 'out of town' school—Evanston Hospital School of Nursing!"

Another student, Karen Waechter, recalls applying to and touring both Michael Reese Hospital School of Nursing and EHSN. When asked how she selected EHSN, she stated, "It is a sweet story. I fell in love with the library at EHSN. I thought the library was very cozy and homelike. It was an easy decision after that."

The book's fourth chapter contains testimony about what life was like for student nurses throughout many decades but highlights student life in the 1970s. This chapter demonstrates the hard work, dedication, and diligence it took to become a nurse. The stories of life in the dormitory will likely be endearing to any diploma nursing graduate and instantly evoke more fond memories. Recent graduates and educators might find some of the stories hard to believe or humorous, and they might even wonder how the students survived. The three years of studying, living, and providing patient care together created lifelong friendships, shared values, and vivid memories. It was "a life worthwhile." Most graduates would not trade those three years at EHSN for any other type of education.

Readers of the fourth chapter will learn about the bonds that students formed by living and studying in the same dormitory. The memories span from late-night studying to celebrating milestones with other students. Kathryn Gray, who started her nursing education at EHSN in 1969, stated, "There is lots to remember . . . but primarily I made lifelong friends with other women in the dorm. Sue, Beth, Deb, and I still spend at least one weekend a year together at Sue's house in Chicagoland. During COVID, we had Zoom meetings together every Monday." After browsing this chapter, the reader will hopefully want to contact their classmates to reconnect and rehash their nursing school memories.

The fifth and final chapter explores how graduation from EHSN was merely the beginning of a life as a nurse. The chapter's title reflects how students never gave up and how they proudly carried the values and skills they learned in nursing school throughout their lives. It highlights some students' experiences on their graduation day—June 17, 1972—and descriptions of their lives over the next 50 years. For Karen Waechter, graduation day was personal; her father, Bill Jones, gave the commencement speech, ending it by saying, "With love, Dad."

Many of the 1972 graduates completed additional education. Some remained at Evanston Hospital to begin their careers and later continued nursing at different healthcare facilities. One graduate, Barbara Ann McQuillan, stayed at Evanston Hospital for her entire 48-year nursing career. The majority of graduates worked as bedside nurses. Some taught nursing, conducted healthcare research, or became leaders and consultants in the healthcare field. Others used their skills to build diverse careers outside the healthcare industry, like Roberta Hilliger, who owned a radio station. Many graduates moved out of the Chicagoland area, and some returned back to their hometowns.

Exploring how EHSN graduates led their lives verifies that diploma schools of nursing prepared graduates by giving them the skills and education they needed to craft a meaningful life in providing patient care. Fifty years later, most graduates had cared for or were caring for family members or close friends with healthcare challenges. The nursing skills they learned never went unused as they helped many navigate the healthcare system. But even more important than the skills the diploma nursing programs provided were the values they taught, which prepared graduates to contribute to society and lead a life with a framework of caring.

Nursing conversations in the 1960s and 1970s centered around how and where nurses should be educated. The choices were a hospital-based program or a nursing program housed in an academic setting. These discussions led to a lot of thoughtful reflection and some divisiveness. As hospital-based educational programs were becoming more costly, technology was evolving, new teaching methods were being developed, and patient care was growing more complex and specialized. It was believed that nurses needed a more general liberal arts education along with learning specific nursing skills to excel in their professional and personal lives. As these conversations evolved, diploma schools of nursing started to fade away as most of them closed, became affiliated with universities, or started their own colleges.

In 1984, after 86 years of educating nurses, EHSN closed. The authors of this book are hoping that diploma nursing programs will be cherished, diploma nurses will be respected, and both the schools and the nurses will be remembered in history.

If you are a diploma graduate, the authors hope that by reading this book and viewing its lively images, you will be brought back to your own cherished memories of classmates, study times, clinical learning, instructor moments, adored patients, and the pride that came with graduating as a nurse—a diploma nurse. Perhaps the book will even enliven your senses of feel, smell, and touch as your mind draws on your own recollection of this rich time in your life. We expect you to laugh, remember, and perhaps cry while reading the book. If you are a more recent nursing graduate or nursing instructor, we hope you will find some of this history interesting and of value. We know you will find some of these stories unimaginable.

Evanston Hospital School of Nursing: 1898–1984 was initially conceived as a gift to the EHSN class of 1972. But in reality, this book is a gift to all nurses, because it preserves a special time in our nursing education history. The authors invite you to relive and cherish your memories and be part of nursing history. Please tell your nursing education story and search for your own nursing school pictures from years ago, helping to make your story come alive and become part of diploma nursing school history.

One

A Time for Us
EHSN in the Beginning

Evanston Emergency Hospital, the first hospital in the Village of Evanston, was originally housed in an eight-room cottage. The building's transformation from cottage to hospital was complete by 1893. The Benevolent Society, an Evanston ladies' association, believed that care of the sick needed to be moved from the home to hospitals. A cottage was bought for $4,300 in 1891, during a typhoid and smallpox outbreak.

By 1898, the hospital had a new location on Ridge Avenue with 18 beds, owned a horse-drawn ambulance, and had been renamed Evanston Hospital. That same year, it established a two-year diploma nursing program called the Evanston Training School for Nurses, to both educate students and provide trained staff for patient care. The school graduated its first two nurses in 1901.

Dr. Sarah Brayton, a medical staff member, was instrumental in gaining approval of the nursing school by stating, "Nursing is no longer a mere vocation . . . but a powerful force in the world's welfare. . . . Scientific training, resulting in methods, accuracy and the attainment of technical knowledge has elevated the work of the nurse from ignorant inaccuracy to a skilled profession."

The first classes contained no more than six students, set high teaching standards, and admitted only women with high purpose and character. The hospital was determined to have a model school in connection with its model hospital.

The school's purpose, as outlined in 1898, was "to give young women entering the school the best possible preparation for the nursing profession, whether they serve in private, institutional or public health fields." The two-year nursing program consisted of days that included more than 14 hours of work and instruction, with students reporting for clinical duty on their second day of training. The days included 12 hours of providing clinical care and at least two hours of lectures. The school became a three-year nursing program in 1906.

By 1909, the school had held its first formal graduation ceremony, and in 1910, it had its first residence building, Patten Hall. Evanston Hospital had grown to become a 250-bed teaching hospital and was contributing to medical research by 1920. At the same time, the school of nursing was also growing and changing. In 1909, the school established a relationship with Northwestern University, and by 1913 the nursing students graduated with a degree alongside other Northwestern students followed by a pinning ceremony at the hospital where they recieved their diplomas. In 1923, Evanston Training School for Nurses became known as Evanston Hospital School of Nursing.

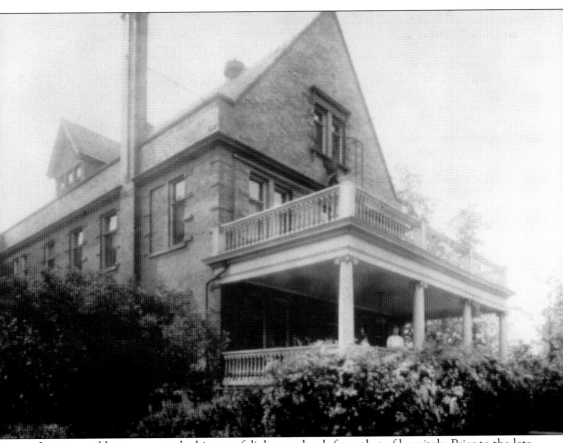

It is impossible to separate the history of diploma schools from that of hospitals. Prior to the late 1880s, nursing care was usually provided in the home by elderly, inexperienced women or women of religious orders. With hospitals starting to emerge, there was a need for trained staff. The hospitals created nursing schools to train students and staff their hospitals. Evanston Emergency Hospital is pictured here.

Rebecca N. Butler and Maria Huse Wilder of the Benevolent Society believed patients needed to be cared for by trained individuals in a hospital rather than in private homes. With the assistance of Dr. Merritt Bragdon (pictured), they raised funds to support Evanston Emergency Hospital.

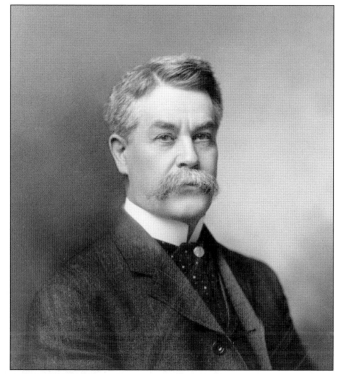

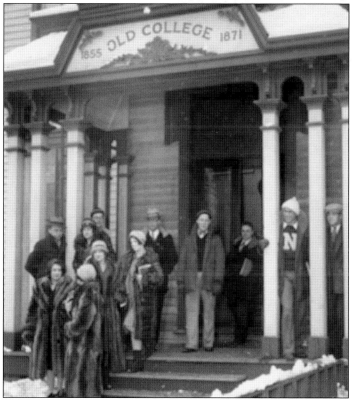

In the early 1900s, Evanston Hospital expanded and became a teaching hospital. Louis W. Sauer developed a vaccine for whooping cough at Evanston Hospital in the 1920s. A toxin for the prevention of scarlet fever was also developed there. In 1920, Evanston Hospital had 250 beds. By the 1930s, it had become a respected research center. The hospital and nursing school had affiliations with Northwestern University, pictured here. (Archives of Northwestern University.)

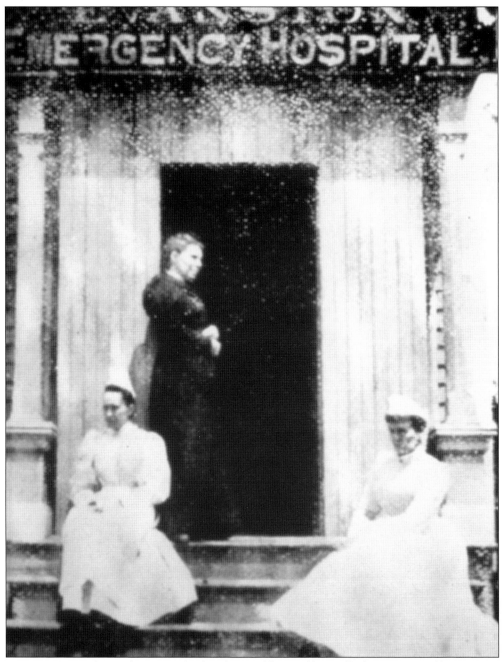

Evanston Hospital treated patients whether they could or could not afford care. Eventually, Evanston had two other hospitals: St. Francis Hospital, which opened in 1901, and Evanston Sanitarium, later renamed Community Hospital of Evanston, which opened in 1914 and closed in 1980.

Evanston Hospital grew by enlarging the number of beds, building new hospital sites, or acquiring and partnering with other hospitals. The hospital also started centers of excellence. In 1981, the hospital developed the Kellogg Cancer Center. It was the first community hospital in the nation to do so. Today, the hospital is part of NorthShore University HealthSystem.

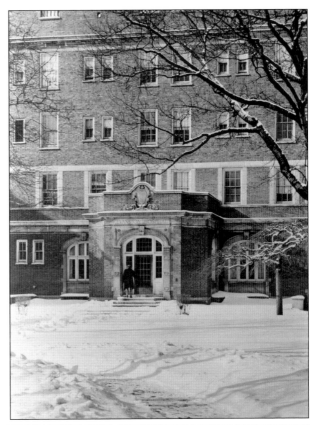

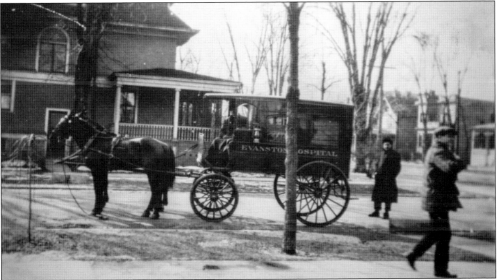

Prior to the late 19th century, nurses were not really trained and certainly not trained with similar standards. During the American Civil War, over 2,000 women enlisted to care for the wounded. They did not have training or knowledge of how to care for the wounded. They did not practice handwashing or isolation. This image shows Evanston Emergency Hospital's ambulance in its early years.

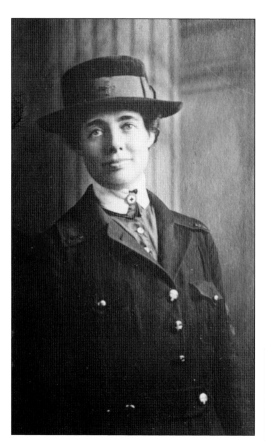

Formal education for nurses started at the end of the 19th century, during the Civil War and the Industrial Revolution. These events led to the recognition of a need for nurses to be professionally trained. Florence Nightingale is credited with developing a model for educating nurses. (Library of Congress.)

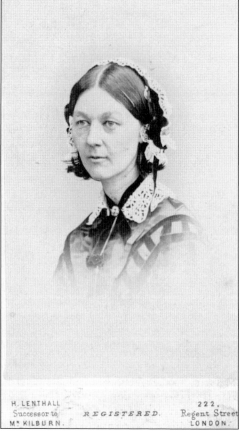

In 1872, New England Hospital for Women and Children became the first school in the United States to offer a formal training program. It offered a one-year curriculum, with 12 hours of lectures. Students were taught how to take vital signs and apply bandages. This photograph features Florence Nightingale, who is considered the founder of nursing education. (Library of Congress.)

H. LENTHALL
Successor to
M.ª KILBURN.

REGISTERED.

222,
Regent Street
LONDON.

Student nurses in 1872 were not allowed to know the names of the medications they gave to patients—the medication bottles were labeled by numbers. Pictured are nurses working in a hospital. Their caps were a symbol of their nursing school and were used for grooming purposes. EHSN had four different caps, with the final one designed in 1971.

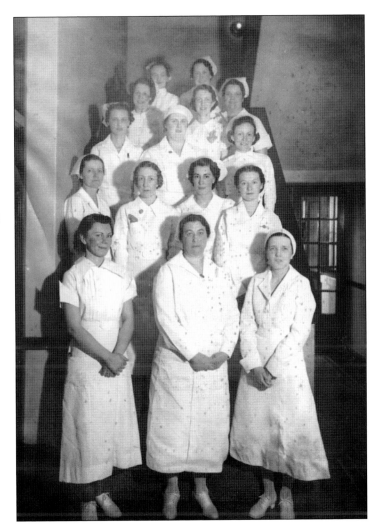

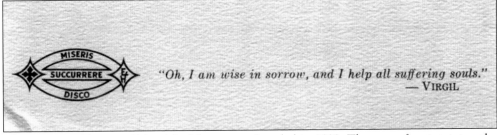

"Oh, I am wise in sorrow, and I help all suffering souls."
— Virgil

The Evanston Training School for Nurses was founded in 1898. The cost of maintaining the school that year was $1,484. The nursing pin pictured here at left was designed by faculty in 1901 after they rejected commissioned pin designs created by Chicago jewelers. This pin was awarded to the first two graduates in 1901 and to the school's final graduates in 1984. It features the school motto, *Miseris Sucurrere Disco*, a quote from Virgil that roughly translates to, "I learn to succor the unfortunate" or "I learn to help those in need." (Barbara McQuillan.)

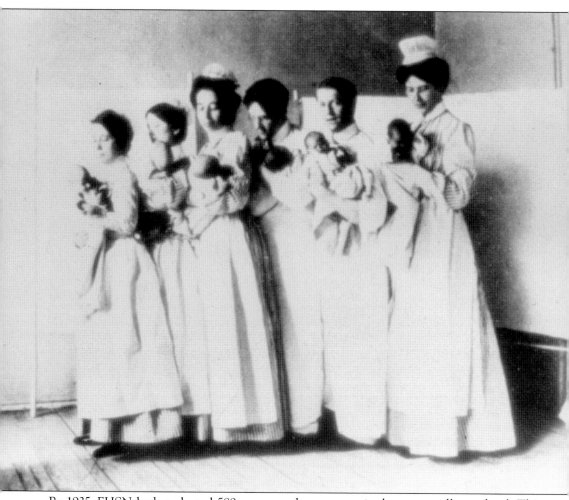

By 1935, EHSN had graduated 589 nurses and was recognized as an excellent school. This photograph shows student nurses in the Evanston Hospital maternity ward in 1907.

Two

MORNING HAS BROKEN
THE STORY OF EHSN

The Nightingale School of Nursing, founded in 1860, was a model for diploma nursing schools in teaching the foundations and principles of nursing knowledge and skills. Anna Locke, a nursing graduate from Blockley Hospital, was the first nursing superintendent of Evanston Hospital, and her job included the duty of being the director of the Evanston Training School for Nurses. Locke was educated by Alice Fisher, who was trained by Florence Nightingale at St. Thomas Hospital in London.

Many nursing programs abandoned the Nightingale training model to be more service-oriented in providing care to patients. Curricula were not standardized, and students had very little classroom time. The students performed free labor while learning hands-on nursing care. Eventually, nursing education focused on not only providing care but also on learning the basics of the profession.

Evanston Training School for Nurses started a two-year program in 1898 and graduated the first two nurses in 1901. The school converted to a three-year program in 1906. Students worked lengthy days and provided patient care starting on the second day of their training. In 1909, the school affiliated with Northwestern University and eventually became a combined nursing university program, making it one of the first baccalaureate programs in the country for nurses. Student nurses graduated with Northwestern students, then participated in a pinning ceremony at the hospital. Nursing students' electives remained at Northwestern University after the closing of the combined program in the 1960s.

Mildred Newton, a 1924 EHSN graduate, was the commencement speaker at the school's 1964 graduation. She said, "Change is the mark of a good school, for only schools which are not static will incorporate new developments in the field of medicine, nursing and education." Her comment was made 20 years before the school closed in 1984.

During the tenure of the school, student nurses lived and studied in five different locations in addition to the campus of Northwestern University: Evanston Hospital's administration building (1898), the Cable Building (1900), Patten Hall (1910), Patten Memorial Hall (1930), and Kendell College Campus (1975). EHSN's training locations, living quarters, curricula, faculty qualifications, student rules, uniforms, and caps all changed over time, but the nursing pin remained the same.

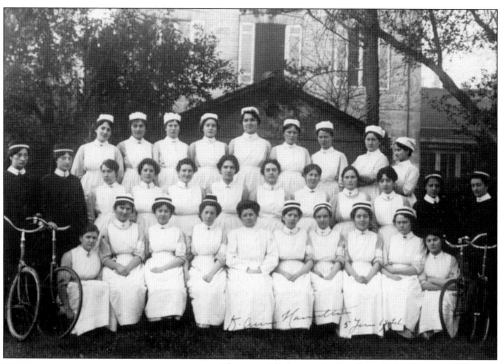

Florence Nightingale developed the first model of nursing education, teaching both the scientific knowledge behind nursing and the "how" of providing care. She believed that education was necessary to "teach not only what is to be done but how to do it . . . and the whys of such thing being done." Anna Locke is credited with developing the excellent Florence Nightingale standards that lasted throughout the history of EHSN. The 1921 graduating class of the Florence Nightingale School is pictured here in Bordeaux, France. (Library of Congress.)

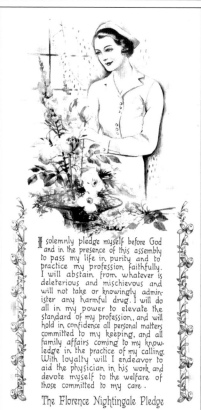

I solemnly pledge myself before God and in the presence of this assembly to pass my life in purity and to practice my profession faithfully. I will abstain from whatever is deleterious and mischievous and will not take or knowingly administer any harmful drug. I will do all in my power to elevate the standard of my profession, and will hold in confidence all personal matters committed to my keeping, and all family affairs coming to my knowledge in the practice of my calling. With loyalty will I endeavor to aid the physician in his work and devote myself to the welfare of those committed to my care.

The Florence Nightingale Pledge

Formal education for nurses started in the United States at the end of the 19th century. During both the Civil War and the Industrial Revolution, it was recognized that nurses needed to be trained. The Nightingale Pledge was recited during the candle-lighting ceremony at most nursing diploma schools—and certainly at EHSN. (Carolyn Smeltzer.)

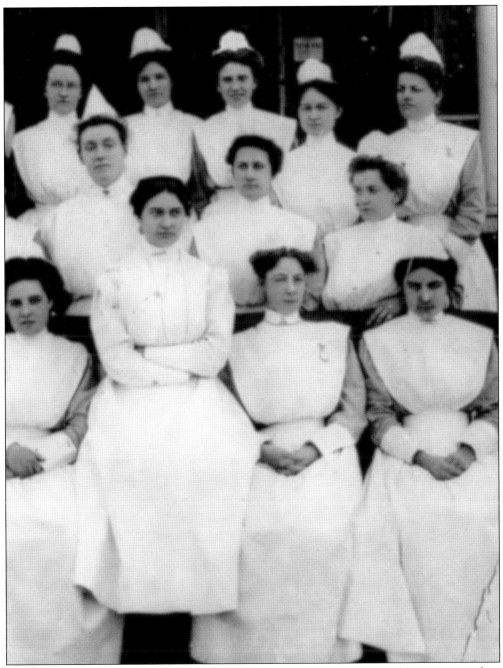

EHSN provided women with an education at a reasonable cost, while the students were providing nursing care to hospitalized patients. EHSN student nurses are pictured here in the early 1900s with their instructors. The instructors are in all white, while the students are wearing blue-striped uniforms overlaid with a white apron.

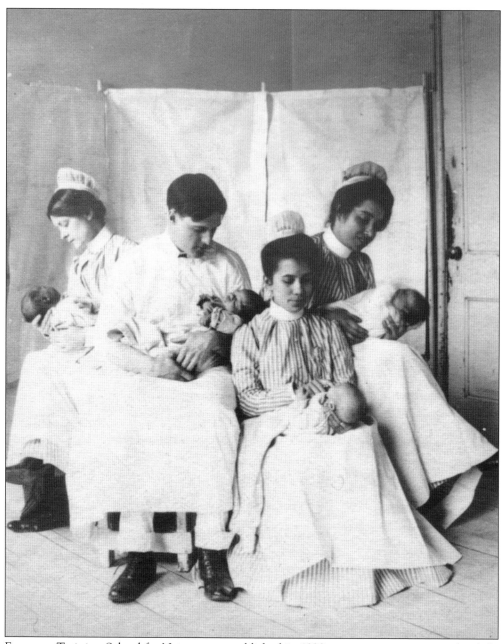

Evanston Training School for Nurses was established in 1898 as a two-year training school. In 1901, the first graduates were Annie L. Carter and Sarah J. Elliott. In the early years, no more than six students were admitted to each class due to limited space and teachers. By 1948, EHSN had graduated 1,157 nurses.

Anna Locke, the first nursing superintendent at Evanston Training School for Nurses, was responsible for both the hospital nursing department and the school. By 1904, hospital leadership had separated the duties of the nursing superintendent into two positions—one for the hospital's nursing department and the other for the school of nursing.

The superintendent of nurses reported to the hospital board. Her duty was to train the students with accurate scientific knowledge. Classes were taught after nursing care was performed in the hospital. The superintendent was responsible for maintaining proper decorum and discipline among the nurses. Here, a student nurse is pictured with a new mother and her baby.

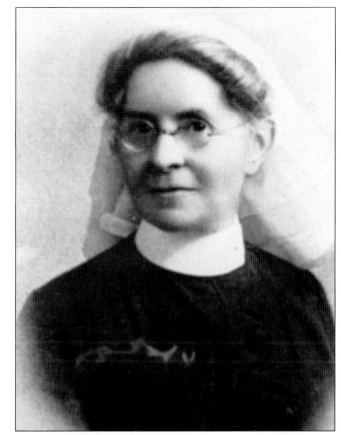

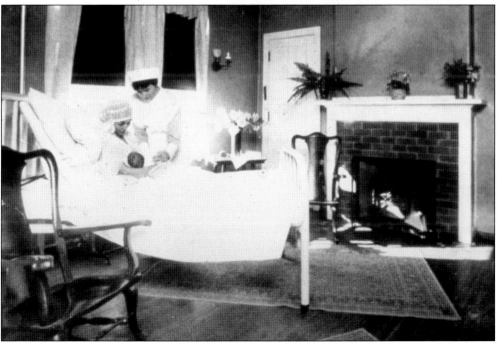

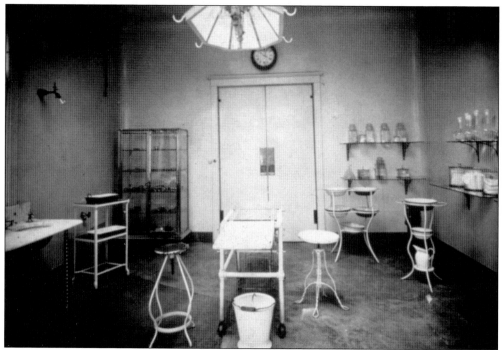

In 1904, Anna Locke was named supervisor of the hospital. The graduating students were rewarded $100 for the care they gave during training, and the students did not have to pay tuition. In 1907, students started to receive a stipend of $5 per month to replace the $100 at graduation. Pictured is an early procedural room at Evanston Emergency Hospital.

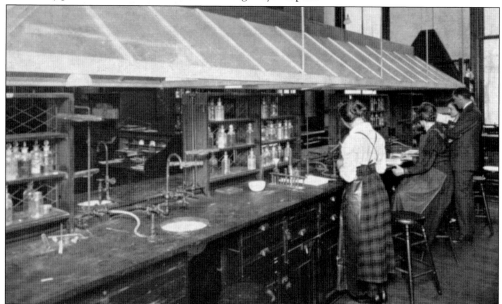

Evanston Hospital, as well as the training school for nurses, was under the jurisdiction of the board of directors. Early in the school's history, a special training school committee was formed. The committee's duties were to cooperate with the superintendent and report the school's progress and needs. These nursing students are pictured in Northwestern University's laboratory.

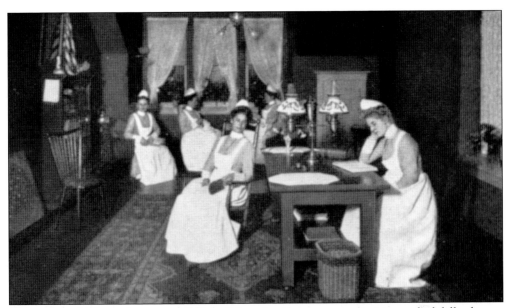

The students had specific accountabilities. They signed a contract promising to faithfully observe and comply with all rules and regulations of the school and hospital. They agreed to remain in the program for two years (or three years, starting in 1906) and observe as well as follow the teachings of instructors. Students had a one-month probation period after they were accepted into the school. Some students are shown here studying in the Cable Building.

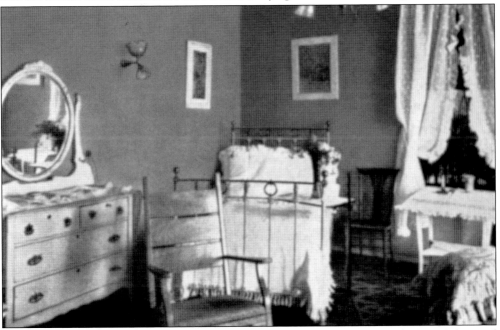

The "Contract for Pupil Nurses, Evanston Training School for Nurses," stated: "I ... understand the rules and regulations imposed, and in consideration of the advantages offered by the Evanston Hospital Training School for Nurses, do hereby agree to remain a pupil for a period of two years . . . to obey the teaching and direction of those in authority over me." This contract was discontinued in 1913. This image features a typical student room in the administrative building.

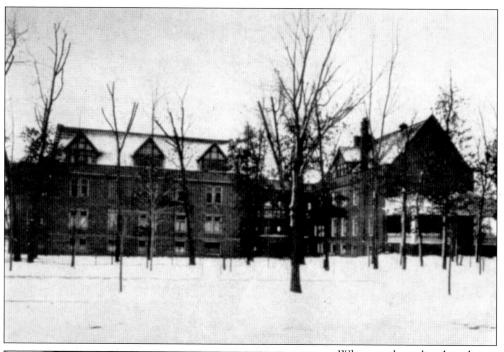

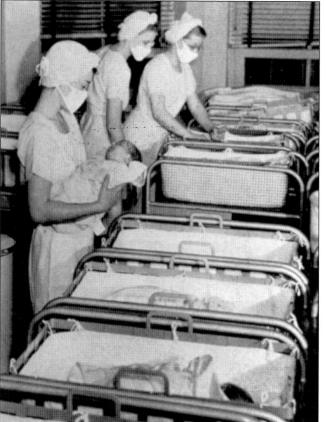

When students lived in the administrative building, they were also scattered in the hospital. They had a dining room in the basement and a sitting area on the first floor. In the Cable (pictured) and Williams Buildings, students had sleeping rooms on the third floor and a larger "gathering room" used for teaching, studying, and socializing.

From 1898 to 1906, the school program was two years long; it later evolved into a three-year diploma program that included four months of maternity nursing. The 1910 Illinois Nurse Practice Act required that schools meet specific qualifications, including teaching maternity nursing.

The first building designated for nurses was Patten Hall, which was built in 1909. James Patten (pictured) asked how many rooms were needed, and the answer was 25. He doubled the number of rooms, noting that the hospital and school were growing.

Patten Hall was a gift from James A. Patten in memory of his brother George. James Patten and his wife, Amanda, contributed to the second nurses' residence building, Patten Memorial Hall, in 1930. These students are making a four-corner bed with a dummy patient in Patten Hall.

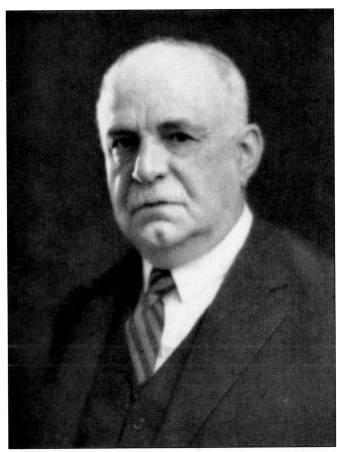

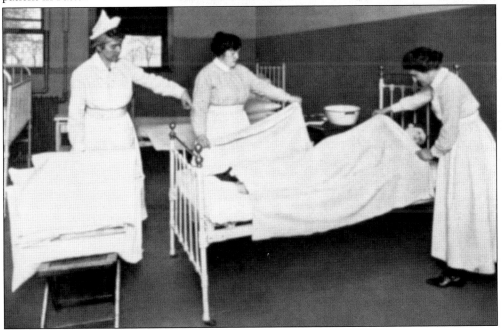

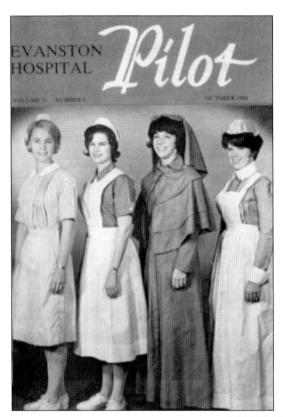

EVANSTON HOSPITAL *Pilot*

VOLUME 5   NUMBER 5   OCTOBER 1966

Simple cotton dresses were the student uniforms during the probation period. After probation, they were given indoor and outdoor uniforms. The indoor blue-striped uniform (far right) had long sleeves with a bishop's collar and a white apron that almost reached the floor. The cap was not washable and was replaced as needed. The outdoor uniform (second from right) was a long grey coat and a hat with a long veil. The indoor uniform changed four times, as did the cap, during EHSN's existence.

By the time EHSN closed in 1984, the dress code included a pantsuit made of the same fabric as the dress uniform. The student could wear either when providing care. From the beginning, the school uniform was always blue-and-white-striped.

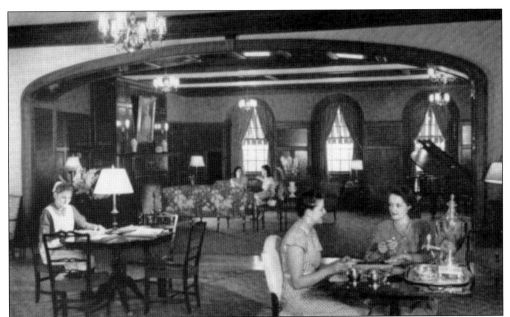

Dedication to nursing was the foremost responsibility of the nursing students. They had strict curfews and could only receive guests on weekends. Patten Memorial Hall's living room had tiny open cubbyholes where students could entertain guests. Eventually, with permission from her parents, a student could have male visitors in her room on Sunday afternoons. The reception area was also used for tea time.

The Illinois Nurse Practice Act of 1910 defined the standards required for school accreditation. Evanston Training School for Nurses received certification in 1912. The school always met all standards for regulatory requirement, including the Nurse Cadet Program. Prior to Evanston Hospital having a maternity ward, the students studied at the Chicago Lying-in Hospital. This 1927 letter was sent to an expectant mother.

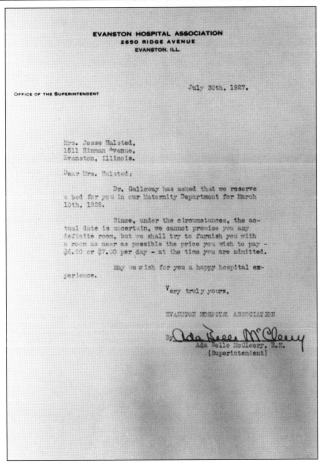

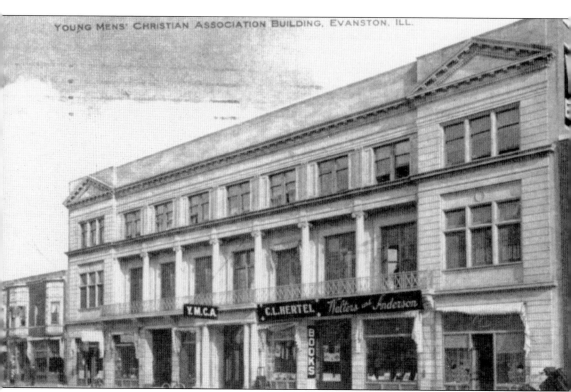

The first public formal commencement of the Evanston Training School for Nurses was held on June 17, 1909, at Evanston's YMCA building in the Women's Club Room. Prior to this, the students did not have a graduation ceremony. The YMCA in Evanston—now the McGaw YMCA—was established in 1885. In 1898, it moved to Orrington Avenue. This is the building where the 1909 graduates held their ceremony. (Archives of McGaw YMCA.)

Cady Mcquire, a 1909 Evanston Training School for Nurses graduate, commented, "It was such a happy day. Miss Locke and Miss Bird, all aflutter, making certain that each of us in the graduating class had our clean cap on at the right angle, that our uniforms were perfect, and entreating us to behave with proper decorum . . . we each carried a bouquet. We felt so proud." Pictured here are Anna Locke (left), nursing superintendent, and Edith Bird, director of the school.

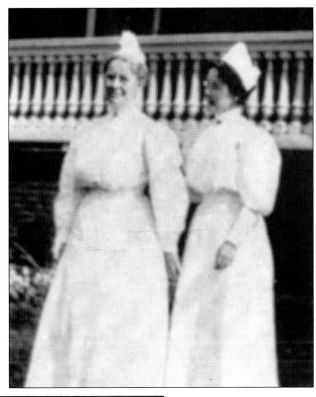

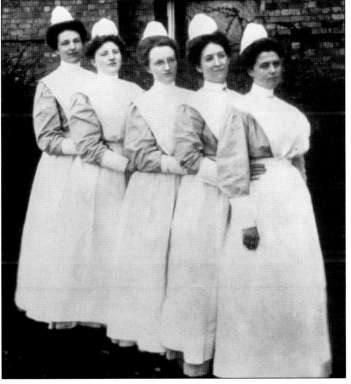

The first class graduated two nurses in 1901— Annie Carter and Sarah Elliott. The class of 1902 also had two graduates. The class of 1909 had eight. In that year, Anna Locke and Edith Bird left Evanston Hospital, but their influence of maintaining high standards remained. Helen Bloomfield became directress of nurses in 1910 and served in the position until 1914. Pictured are student nurses in the early 1900s.

33

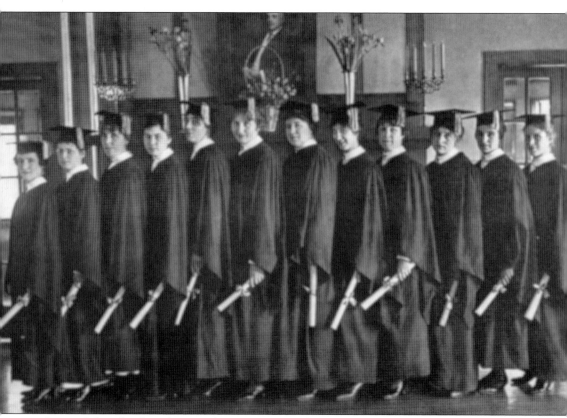

Some of the school's milestones between 1912 and 1913 included accreditation by the Illinois State Board of Nurse Examiners, student night duty being shortened from 12 hours to 10, and students learning about infectious diseases in the hospital's Contagious Disease Center. The last graduation on the Patten lawn was held on June 18, 1912. In 1913, students started graduating at Northwestern University, followed by a pinning ceremony in Patten Hall. This is the class of 1917.

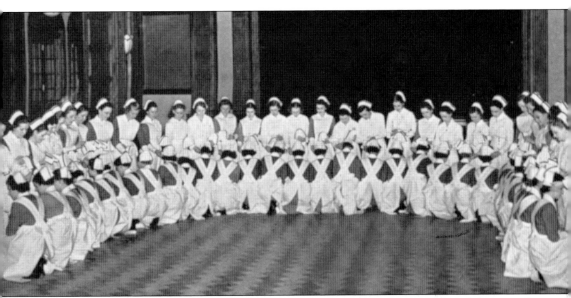

In 1915, the Evanston Training School for Nurses students and faculty created a celebration of capping called a black band ceremony. The bands on the caps indicated the students' year of study. The first event had music and a speech, as reported in the Nurse Bulletin in 1915. The capping ceremony continued throughout the school's existence. This black band capping ceremony was for the class of 1939.

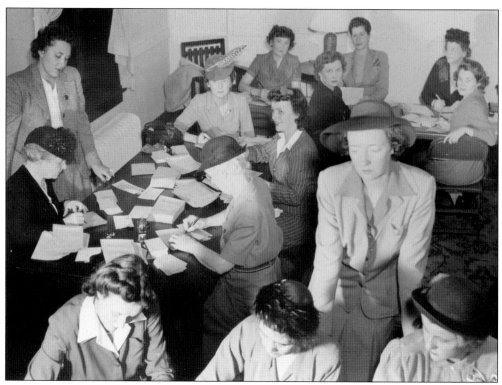

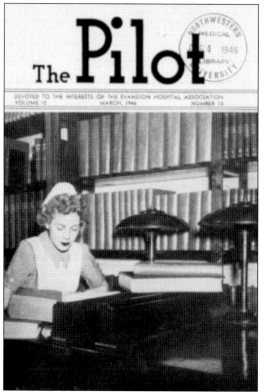

The Pilot

DEVOTED TO THE INTERESTS OF THE EVANSTON HOSPITAL ASSOCIATION
VOLUME 10   MARCH, 1946   NUMBER 10

The training school had an affiliation with Children's Memorial Hospital in Chicago prior to Evanston Hospital having a children's ward. Children's Memorial had a nursing diploma program until 1924 and sent students to Evanston Hospital to learn adult nursing care. Pictured are volunteers putting together the mailing for the *Pilot*, the hospital's journal that frequently featured the school's activities along with hospital news.

In 1926, EHSN students had to take an Otis Test, commonly used to measure intelligence. The school called this "a mental alertness test." Students began to pay for their educations in 1927. Tuition was $375.50 in 1932—including education, uniforms, books, healthcare, and testing. The school had a library (pictured on the cover of this March 1946 issue of the *Pilot*) from its beginning in 1898.

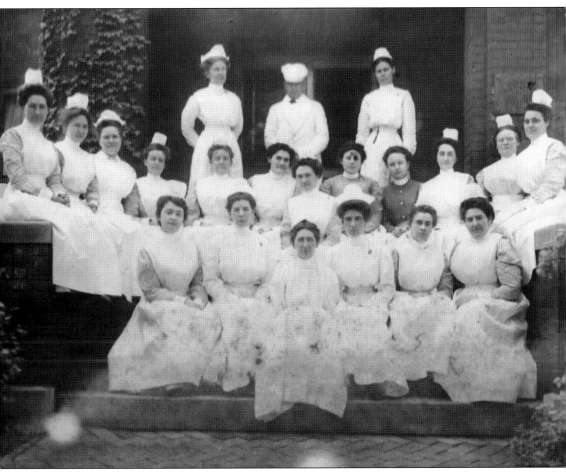

By 1911, the school's curriculum included 334 hours of theory. EHSN had graduated 589 nursing students by 1935, and 1,157 by 1948. At this time, diploma nursing programs were producing the majority of the nation's nurses. EHSN provided women with education at a reasonable cost, while the students provided nursing care. This photograph shows students with Anna Locke and Edith Bird.

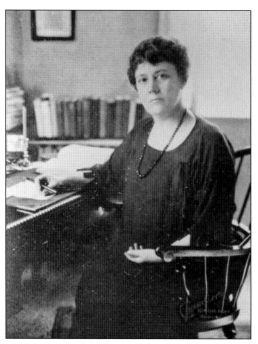

Ada Belle McCleery was directress of the training school from 1915 through 1921, then became the hospital's first female administrator, serving in that position until her retirement in 1941. She spent two months traveling and evaluating other nursing school programs before creating a vision, curriculum, and mission for the Evanston Training School for Nurses.

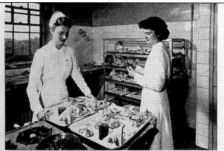

A nurse and Miss Braley in a floor kitchen during the serving period.*

counter the girl in charge of salads has prepared and lined up the requested number for G 2; nearby are grouped the salads for G 3; and farther along, those for G 4. Other items of the menu are being placed by individual servings in regular positions in the kitchen where they will be picked up and placed on the giant cart which goes to each floor. In the special diet kitchen, food for diabetic trays, reduction menus, etc., is being prepared to go along with the regular food to the floor where it has been requested.

Beginning at eleven o'clock each morning, a parade of carts takes the food to the many small kitchens where it is popped into refrigerators or placed in steam tables. In each of

[10] THE PILOT

these kitchens a dietary employee is responsible for serving the food attractively and a nurse in charge checks out each patient's tray to make sure that he receives the proper menu.

Like the medical departments of the Hospital, the Dietary Department is also a teaching organization. Student nurses spend six weeks in the special diet kitchen, where they prepare food for therapeutic diets under supervision and learn to weigh it when necessary. This practical experience follows classroom and laboratory instruction in nutrition, diet and disease—a total of sixty hours—presented by members of the Dietary Staff.

Miss Danahay and Miss Kirby

also instruct Hospital patients in special diet preparation. When such a diet has been requested by the doctor, one of these dietitians calls on the patient to work out a dietary program within the limits allowed, and also in many cases teaches the patient or his parents or relatives how to manage the diet after the return home.

In two clinics a week in the Outpatient Department, Miss Kirby plans prescribed diets with patients. In the Diabetic Clinic, she may teach the patient or relatives how to manage it. In the Nutrition Clinic, she also works with nutritional prob-

lems, such as that of the overweight or underweight patient, the patient who requires a low sodium diet, or special diets prescribed for children.

The Dietary Department is called upon to prepare delicacies for special occasions, too—an annual luncheon for graduating nurses, cookies and punch for receptions in Patten Memorial drawing rooms, for dances, etc.

In carrying out their jobs, Miss Colwell pointed out, the members of the Dietary Department work closely with and have the assistance of many other departments. In addition to their close association with the medical and nursing staffs, they

A dietitian instructs students in a Nutrition Laboratory on the preparation of food.*

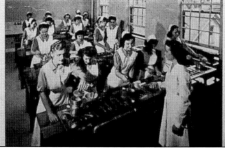

Sarah Corry, an EHSN instructor, wrote a book in 1944 that was dedicated to all nurses "who know but may have forgotten" some of their nursing skills. *Notes on Nursing by a Nurse* was a training book intended to be used as a guide for smaller nursing schools or as a refresher for nurses reentering the field. It was pocket-sized for convenient carrying. This was one of the first nursing books written by an EHSN faculty member.

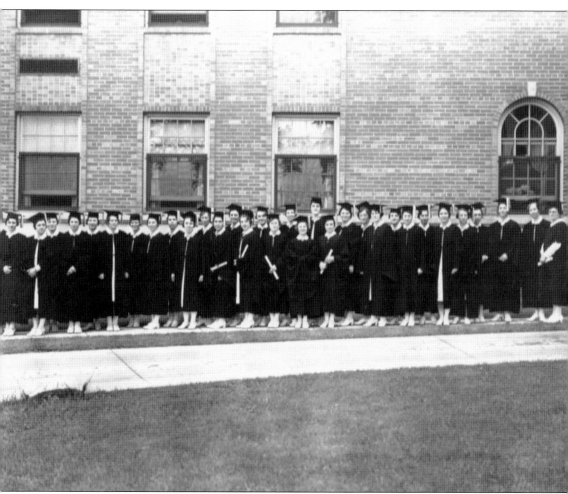

The name of Evanston Training School for Nurses was changed to Evanston Hospital School of Nursing in 1923. This change was significant, as the school was recognized not only for training nurses but also for educating women at Northwestern University. The school offered one of the first bachelor's degree programs in Illinois. Ida B. Smith was the directress of the school from 1921 through 1925.

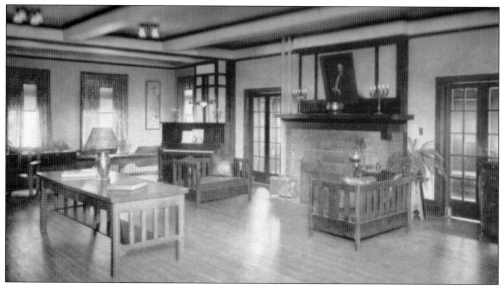

Mildred E. Newton, a 1924 EHSN graduate and dean of Ohio State University, gave the EHSN commencement speech in 1964. As a student, she lived in the Patten Hall residence (pictured).

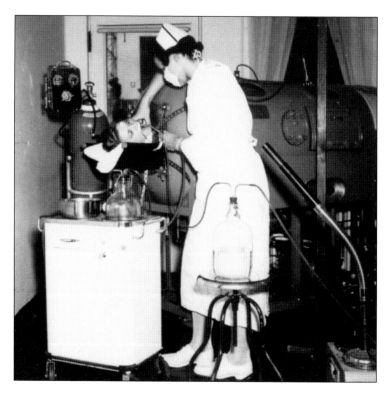

The faculty members at EHSN were always seeking better methods of instruction in the classroom and on the patient care units. The school participated in the National League for Nursing Education's first credentialing process in 1940. EHSN was recognized for having strong standards in student admission, curriculum development, and faculty qualification. This EHSN graduate is providing care to a patient in an iron lung.

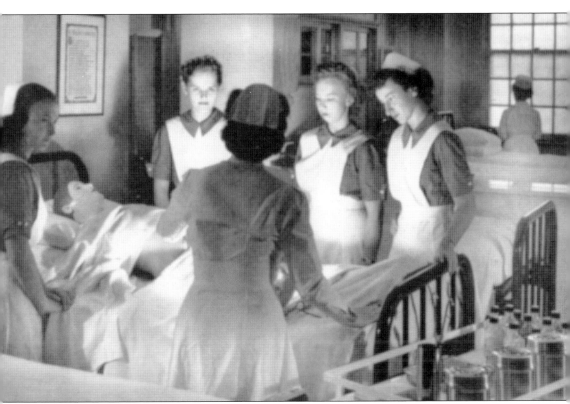

Traditionally, EHSN expected obedience and loyalty from students, who were required to live in the dormitory. When students started living in Patten Memorial Hall in 1930, they had more social activities, including tea receptions, Christmas and Halloween parties, and arranged dances. However, learning nursing skills and theory was always the first priority, as pictured here.

EVANSTON HOSPITAL

Evanston Hospital is a voluntary hospital of approximately 550 beds. Committed first to providing quality patient care and second to a broad educational program, the hospital offers a unique learning environment in a clinical setting that is dynamic and totally patient centered.

EVANSTON HOSPITAL SCHOOL OF NURSING

Founded in 1898, the Evanston Hospital School of Nursing was one of the first schools of professional nursing in Illinois. The school is accredited by the National League for Nursing and holds Title VIII membership in the American Hospital Association.

As a single purpose program for the education of nurses the school has an outstanding faculty, progressive teaching facilities, and provides for nursing experiences in a progressive clinical setting. These factors have consistently contributed to the high standing of the graduates on state board examinations, and in various nursing positions throughout the world.

PHILOSOPHY

The faculty of the Evanston Hospital School of Nursing believes that nursing is a service provided for individuals within a community. This service is concerned with assisting the patient to achieve the highest possible level of physical and mental well-being in his environment. Nursing care involves an understanding of scientific principles basic to nursing and the ability to apply these principles in helping the patient to meet his individual needs.

The faculty believes that the student is an individual and that learning is enhanced by an atmosphere which encourages the development of the student's self awareness, intellectual inquiry, self-direction, creativeness, and maturity. Our nursing program provides an opportunity for the student to develop an understanding of the concepts and principles of nursing. This development requires the application and integration of knowledge from the natural and behavioral sciences and is accomplished by closely correlating classroom instruction with clinical experience in a hospital setting.

It is the faculty's responsibility to prepare the nurse who will become skilled in providing intelligent and thoughtful nursing care. It is emphasized that learning is a continuing process and the student is encouraged to pursue education for professional and personal growth. The graduate of this school should develop a spirit of responsibility as a contributing citizen in a democratic society.

OBJECTIVES

In planning the School curriculum the aim of the faculty is to conduct the student's total learning experience so that the graduate of the School will be able to:

1. Use critical analysis and sound judgment to plan and administer competent nursing care.
2. Establish and maintain effective interpersonal relationships with patients, families, and members of the health team.
3. Contribute to society as a responsible nurse and citizen.

6

According to Helen Dulick, class of 1950, even though more social activities were offered in that period, "It was believed that nurses should be solely devoted to nursing . . . and there wasn't room then for outside activities and interest." She made this statement when she was president of the Evanston Hospital Alumni Association, as quoted in the 1984 *Pilot*. The school's philosophy and objectives in the 1970s are outlined here.

NURSING VI

Pediatric Nursing
Second year — Theory, 80 hours
Lab, 240 hours

Study of the nursing care of the ill child, his hospitalization, and its effects on the child and his family. Includes nursery school experience, observations in a pediatrician's office, and care of children in the outpatient department. Class room instruction includes televised classes.

NURSING VII

Psychiatric Nursing
Third year — Theory, 80 hours
Lab, 240 hours

Study of theoretic knowledge basic to understanding of mental health and illness in order to study the needs of patients with deviations of behavior that interfere with successful adjustment to life. Emphasis is placed on the need for increased understanding of human behavior, a continued development of communications skills, and a deepening awareness of the dynamics of interpersonal relationships. The nurse is also viewed as a member of the community mental health team who has an active responsibility in the prevention, treatment, and rehabilitation of the mentally ill. Classroom instruction includes televised classes.

NURSING VIII

Rehabilitation & Community Nursing
Third year — Theory, 80 hours
Lab, 240 hours

Nursing care of patients with interference in normal motor and/or sensory function. Lab experience is planned to provide for care of patients with orthopedic and neurologic diseases necessitating intensive rehabilitation and utilization of community resources.

NURSING IX

Comprehensive Nursing
Third year — Theory, 80 hours
Lab, 240 hours

Nursing care of patients with complex or multiple nursing care needs. The emphasis is on nursing intervention utilizing advanced nursing knowledge and skills. Applied to care of patients in the emergency room, intensive care unit, coronary care unit and medical-surgical units.

NURSING X

Management of Patient Care
Third year — Theory, 40 hours
Lab, 240 hours

Utilization of principles of leadership, management and supervisory techniques in the role of a team leader. Seminars emphasize problems encountered in team nursing situations that relate to a nurse's responsibility to the patient, to the team, to the institution, and to herself.

NURSING AND THE LAW

Second year — Theory, 15 hours

Study of laws for protection of patients and nurses and the legal implications of nursing functions. Classroom instruction includes televised classes.

HISTORY AND TRENDS IN NURSING

Third year — Theory, 30 hours

Study of current trends in nursing as they have developed from past events. Includes examination of the role of nurses in the community for fostering growth of nursing.

SOCIAL SCIENCES

PSYCHOLOGY

First year, first quarter — Theory, 30 hours

Study of basic concepts of normal human behavior.

SOCIOLOGY

First year, second quarter — Theory, 30 hours

Study of individual behavior in informal, formal groups, and social institutions.

HUMAN DEVELOPMENT I

First year, third quarter — Theory, 40 hours

Study of development of the individual's psychological, sociological, and physiological developmental tasks from adolescence through death.

HUMAN DEVELOPMENT II

Second year, concurrently with Pediatric Nursing — Theory, 30 hours

Study of normal growth and development of children from infancy through adolescence.

COMMUNICATIONS

Second year, fourth quarter — Theory, 20 hours

Study of the language arts with emphasis on dialogue as the key factor in interpersonal relationships.

TYPES OF RELIGIOUS THOUGHT

Second year — Theory, 30 hours

Study of theories and basic concepts of the major religions.

SOCIAL PSYCHOLOGY

Third year — Theory, 30 hours

Study of group formation and group interactions in society.

In 1942, students could spend two years at Rockford College and then three years at EHSN. After completing this five-year program, they graduated with a bachelor of science in nursing (BSN) degree. This is an example of a partial curriculum for students.

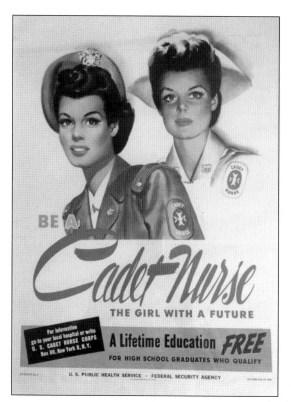

In 1943, EHSN participated in the US Cadet Nurse Corps. The program was created to help alleviate the critical shortage of nurses caused by World War II. The length of instruction was shortened from 36 months to 30 months in order to graduate students sooner. By the 1960s, the school's mission and purpose was refocused on educating local rather than national women in order to meet the healthcare needs of the Evanston community. (Carolyn Smeltzer.)

The EHSN curriculum changed based on the report of the grading committee and the requirements of the US Cadet Nurse Corps. As the curriculum continually evolved, so did the school's admission requirements and the faculty's specialized qualifications. (Carolyn Smeltzer.)

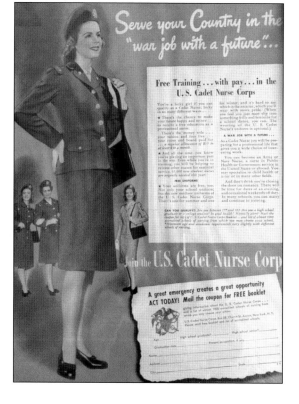

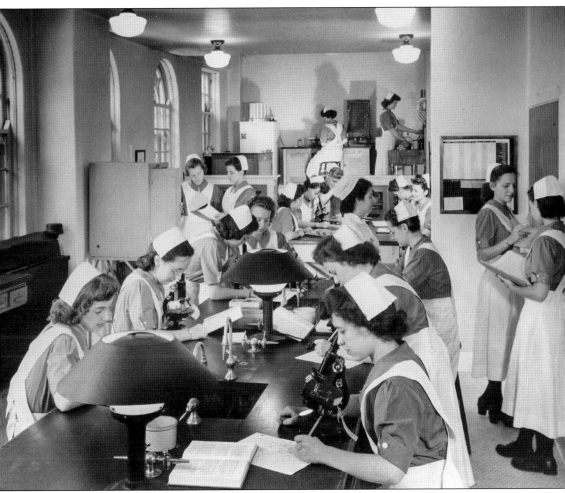

In 1965, EHSN faculty members wrote *Workbook and Study Guide for Medical-Surgical Nursing: A Patient Centered Approach*, published by the C.V. Mosby Company. The book had 20 case studies on how to provide nursing care that ranged in difficulty from simple to complex. It was a critical thinking textbook rather than a rote memory textbook. This book changed nursing education across the country. These students are pictured in Patten Memorial Hall's science laboratory.

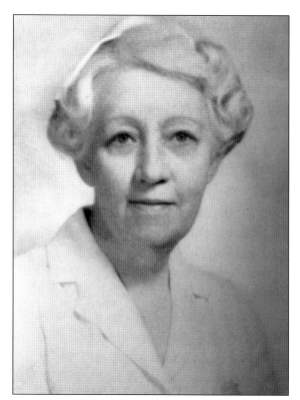

Elizabeth Odell was the longest-running director of EHSN. She was a graduate of Montreal General Hospital School of Nursing and McGill School of Graduate Nursing. She served in the Canadian Army Medical Corps during World War I and received the Royal Red Cross, First Class. She retired after 26 consecutive years of service, from 1925 to 1951. Odell is credited with guiding the school through many positive changes.

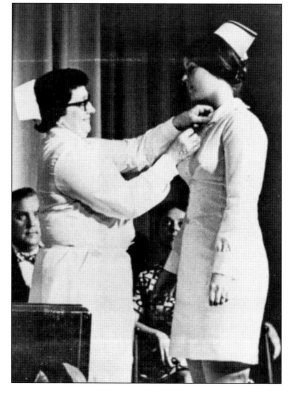

In 1965, EHSN was part of the 17-area nursing school project used to assist in teaching rural nursing students. The Chicago Video Nursing program used a television channel to broadcast teaching videos. Dorothy Johnson, director of EHSN from 1959 to 1966, served as chairman of the council responsible for producing the videos. June Werner, who was chairperson of the nursing department from 1971 through 1990, is shown pinning a nursing graduate. (Carolyn Smeltzer.)

In 1967, the school initiated an open curriculum. By 1971, the school had a teaching system of student driven learning. Education and testing were done with a slideshow presentation. The National League of Nursing described the program as "an educational approach designed to accommodate the learning needs and career goals of the students." Students could learn and test at their own pace. (Barbara McQuillan.)

The school was one of the first, if not *the* first, to have individual self-learning classes. The curriculum was centered around the concepts of primary care nursing and care planning. Marjorie Beyers, who served as director of EHSN from 1967 to 1980, was credited with the development of theory-based teaching and independent, self-paced learning. (Family of Marjorie Beyers.)

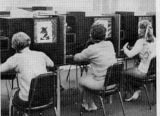

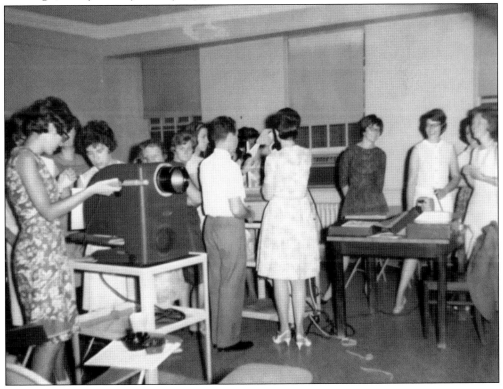

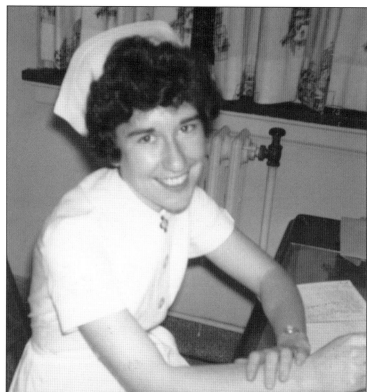

Marjorie Beyers stated: "We were one of the first schools of nursing to drop all barriers to the non-traditional students . . . older people, married women with families, corpsmen from the armed services, and others were welcomed to be a student at EHSN. This was demonstrated by the average age of the nursing student rising." (Family of Marjorie Beyers.)

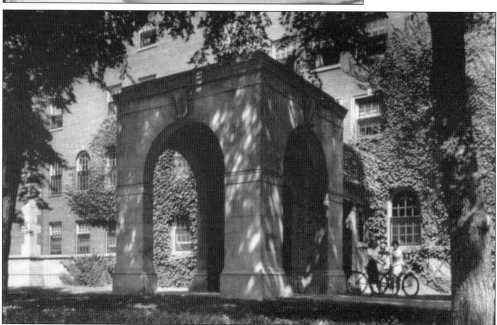

When Patten Memorial Hall was demolished in 1974, it ended a memorable era in EHSN's history. The school of nursing moved to the Kendall College campus. Students had options among study topics and were no longer required to live in the dormitory. The EHSN dormitory property became a parking lot overlooking the golf course.

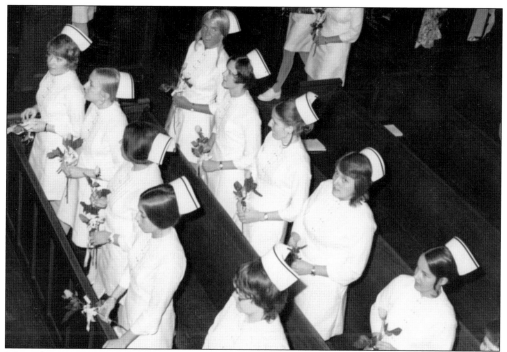

Many discussions and debates were held prior to 1965 as to where and how nursing education should be taught. In that year, the American Nurses Association issued a position statement favoring nursing education to be held in a university. EHSN leadership urged graduates to continue their education after receiving their diplomas. (Family of Marjorie Beyers.)

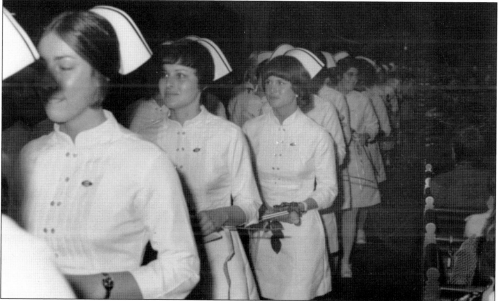

EHSN was closed in 1984 after 86 years of educating nurses. "The demands on nurses to provide highly complex patient care was increasing," stated June Werner, chairperson of Evanston Hospital's nursing department, and "complex patient care required nursing education to be in a university setting." These quotes were reported in the *Pilot* in 1984. (Family of Marjorie Beyers.)

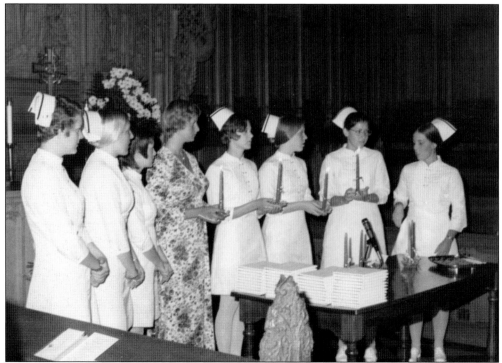

These EHSN students are lighting the candles and reciting the Nightingale Pledge prior to getting pinned and receiving their diplomas. Lighting the candle was representative of Florence Nightingale's nighttime aid to wounded soldiers. The pinning ceremony is symbolic, welcoming the students into nursing, and representative of when Queen Victoria awarded Nightingale the Royal Red Cross in 1855 for her service in the Crimean War. (Family of Marjorie Beyers.)

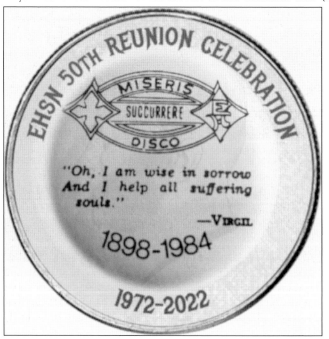

Sarah Brayton and Jessie Bradley designed the EHSN nursing pin after refusing designs provided by Chicago jewelers. The first pins were given to graduates in 1901, and the last were given in 1984, the year the school closed. This EHSN coin was designed for the school's final class in 1984 and restyled for the class of 1972's 50th reunion, which was held in 2022. (Carolyn Smeltzer.)

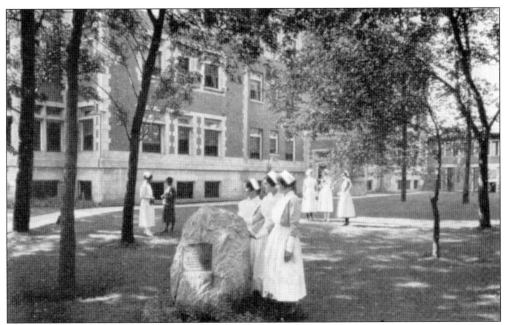

EHSN closed in 1984. June Werner, Evanston Hospital's chairperson of nursing at the time, stated, "This June 1984, the 86-year-old diploma school will close. Today, the technical expertise and scientific knowledge required makes nursing too complex to remain outside the traditional college educational system." Patten Hall is pictured here.

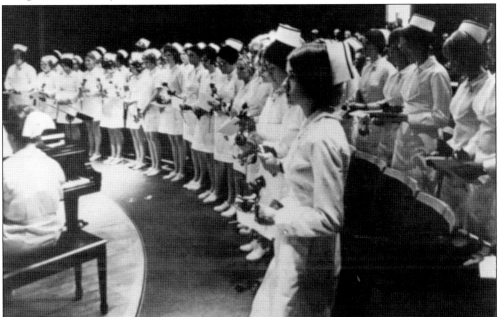

Elizabeth Odell wrote in 1944, forty years before the closing of EHSN, "Nursing students are scattered far and wide. Whether they serve in positions involving great responsibilities, or those of lesser responsibilities, is not vital. The crucial test is not the importance of their positions, but rather the quality of service. The Evanston Hospital School of Nursing has reason to be justly proud of its graduate's service."

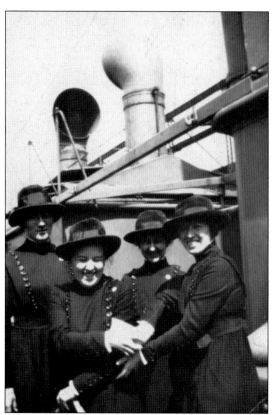

Helen Burnett Wood, a 1914 graduate of EHSN and Northwestern University, volunteered to serve in World War I. She was shot and killed during a practice session on the SS *Mongolia*, which was being used to set up a medical hospital in France. A procession of Red Cross workers, nurses, and Chicago citizens met her body at Union Station and attended her funeral. Pictured are Alice Radcliffe, Ada Crawford, Thelcia Richter, and Helen Wood. (Archives of Northwestern University.)

Helen Burnett Wood is recognized by memorial plaques on the Northwestern University campus, in Evanston Hospital, at Evanston's Patriots Park, and in her hometown in Scotland. Louise Effie Cobe Merwin, a 1924 graduate, was a decorated World War II veteran, pilot, and farmer. At the age of 99, she pinned her grandson's girlfriend, Paige Kubitski, at the 2017 Madonna University graduation. Both nurses are a testimony to Elizabeth Odell's 1944 letter. (Archives of Northwestern University.)

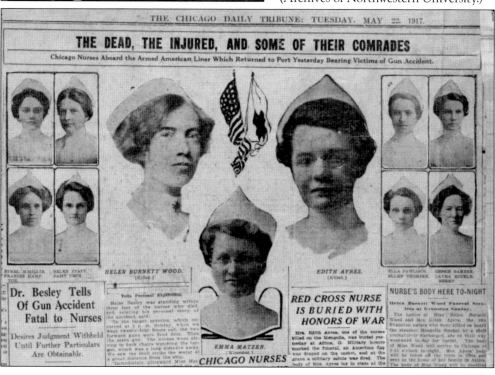

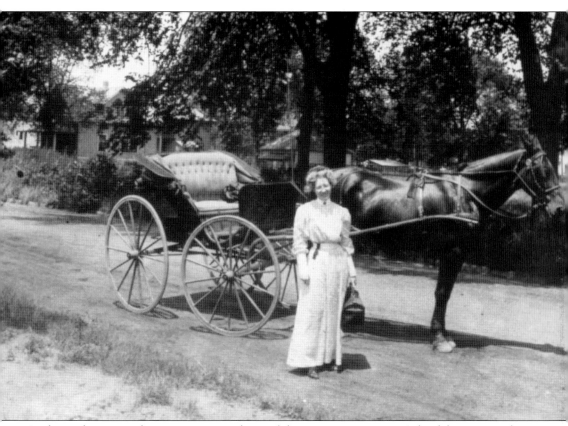

Hedwig Johnson Braden was a 1904 graduate of the Evanston Training School for Nurses. She was the first graduate to become a visiting nurse—another testimony to the words written by Elizabeth Odell in 1944.

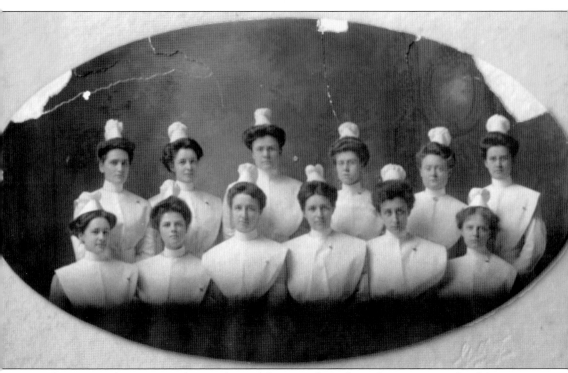

There was only one year when students did not graduate from the Evanston school for nurses, and that was in 1908—due to the school expanding to a three-year program in 1906. An early graduating class of Evanston Training School for Nurses is pictured here.

Three

A PLACE FOR US

MARKETING THE SCHOOL AND SELECTION

The community of Evanston had three hospitals and two nursing school programs in the 1960s: Evanston School of Nursing, created in 1898, and St. Francis School of Nursing, created in 1919. There were numerous other nursing schools in the Chicagoland area. The nation had 1,300 diploma schools of nursing and approximately 7,000 hospitals. By 1960, there were 162 colleges offering a BSN degree, but the diploma schools were still supplying the majority of nurses in the United States.

With more than one in seven hospitals having a school of nursing, it was hard—but not impossible—to differentiate one school from another. Many schools were religiously sponsored, some were affiliated with academic medical centers, and others were associated with community-based hospitals. Some were ethnic-oriented, and a few had educational arrangements with a university. Hospital-based nursing programs wanted to attract local students in hopes they would choose to start their nursing career at the hospital where they trained. The many choices of where a student could study nursing presented a challenge.

EHSN was different than most nursing programs because of its early affiliation with Northwestern University. It was one of the first diploma nursing programs to offer a bachelor's degree along with a nursing diploma. When the college degree was eliminated, students still took their electives at Northwestern University, which was within walking distance of the hospital. Students could earn college credits and experience a college campus while studying nursing courses and skills at the hospital. This was a highlight that distinguished EHSN.

During World War II, EHSN was part of the Cadet Nurse Corps program, which attracted students from across the nation to attend the school. The EHSN faculty were considered national leaders in educational methods and nursing excellence. They shared their knowledge by publishing books and articles. All of these became differentiating factors for EHSN.

The school developed a brochure—"So You Want to Be a Nurse"—in the 1960s to help prospective students determine if they wanted to be a nurse, and if so, why they should select EHSN for their education. The pamphlet's sections included "The Wise Choice," "A Home Community—Near a City," "A Good School," "All Types of Nursing Care," "Pinning and Graduation," "A Happy and Worthwhile Experience," and "Career Opportunities." This marketing material positioned EHSN as "a place for us." In the mid-1970s, EHSN developed a more modern brochure—"The Evanston Hospital School of Nursing, 1975–1977."

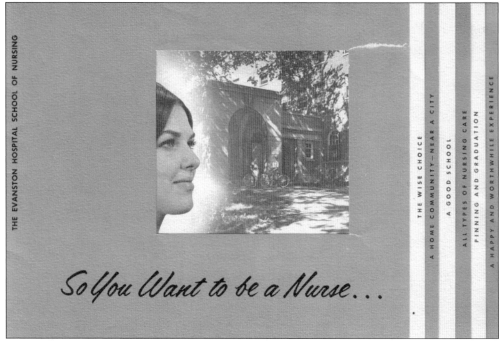

The school's marketing booklet developed in the 1960s highlighted the reasons why one might want to be a nurse as well as why they should choose EHSN. "So You Want to Be a Nurse" was published by EHSN. The booklet was not unusual. In England in the 1960s, one potential nursing student collected over 60 such brochures. Nursing research suggested these advertisements were just "a pretty nurse whose profession was powerless." (Both, Barbara McQuillan.)

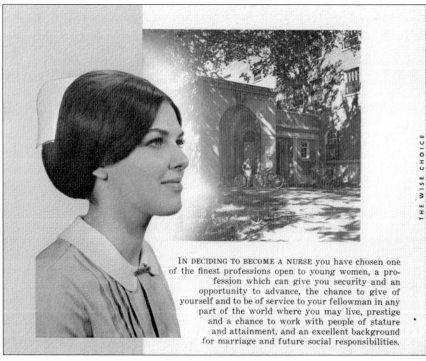

IN DECIDING TO BECOME A NURSE you have chosen one of the finest professions open to young women, a profession which can give you security and an opportunity to advance, the chance to give of yourself and to be of service to your fellowman in any part of the world where you may live, prestige and a chance to work with people of stature and attainment, and an excellent background for marriage and future social responsibilities.

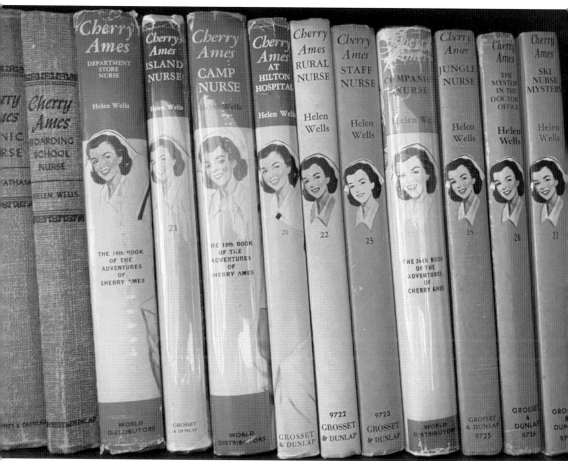

Posters, television programs, movies, and Cherry Ames novels were also used to attract people to the profession of nursing. However, these did not highlight certain schools of nursing. Volunteer opportunities for teenagers to be candy stripers also helped to attract students to the nursing profession. Both authors of this book were candy stripers before becoming nurses. (Robert Hess.)

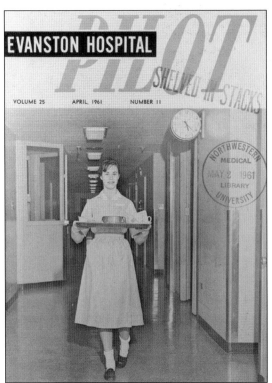

Hospitals organized volunteer opportunities for young girls to become candy stripers in order for them to have an experience of working in a hospital. This cover of the April 1961 issue of the *Pilot* features a candy striper at Evanston Hospital.

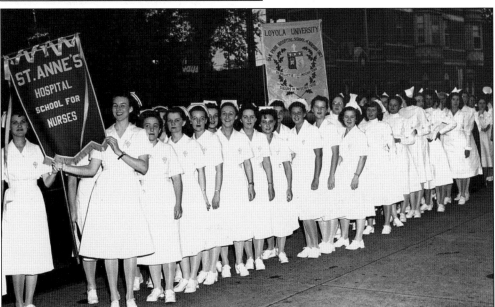

Between 1948 and 1958, Chicago held an annual nurse parade with floats and marchers highlighting and celebrating the work of nurses. The purpose was to attract people to the profession. Merchants, schools of nursing, hospitals, politicians, and religious orders worked together to organize the parade. There could be over 6,000 nurses in the parade and over 100,000 spectators. At the end of the parade, the nurses would gather and renew their nursing vows by reciting the Nightingale Pledge. The parade was Chicago's best-kept secret until *Chicago's Nurse Parade* was published in 2005. (Carolyn Smeltzer.)

The first section of "So You Want to Be a Nurse," titled "The Wise Choice," described why nursing was such a great profession. This section reinforced that the reader had chosen the right career. The entire booklet was focused on nursing being a choice for women. Here, a nursing student poses with a patient and faculty member. (Barbara McQuillan.)

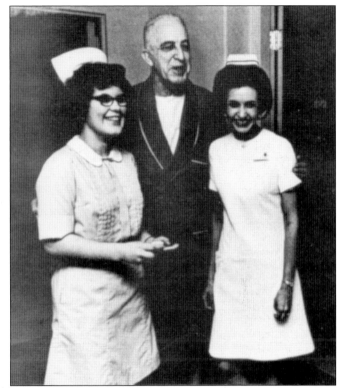

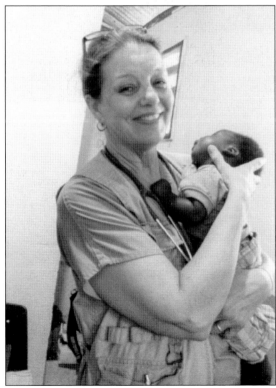

The booklet stated that nursing is "a profession which can give you security and an opportunity to advance," and is also "an excellent background for marriage and future social responsibilities." Kathryn Gray is shown working on the hospital ship *Anastasis* with Mercy Ships in 2007. (Kathryn Gray.)

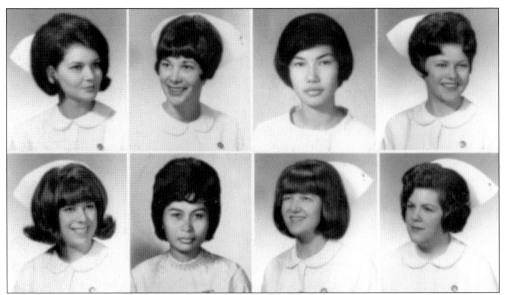

On July 14, 1966, news broke of the murders of eight student nurses and nurses from South Chicago Community Hospital. Author Carolyn Smeltzer was in the Lakeside Veteran's Hospital lounge visiting her sick uncle and overheard angry patients saying, "How could anyone kill a nurse—they help people." These comments reinforced her desire to be a nurse. (Carolyn Smeltzer.)

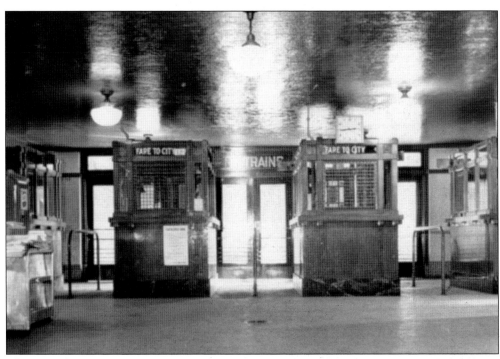

The second section of "So You Want to Be a Nurse," "A Home Community—Near a City," highlighted the location of the school and its activities, which provided both the tranquility of a rural community and the excitement of a big city. Students could use public transportation—the L Purple Line on Central Avenue (pictured)—to travel to the heart of Chicago.

The brochure contained pictures of students at a campfire, on a beach, and at social dances. These mixers were arranged with Great Lakes sailors or Northwestern University fraternities. It was hard to imagine that just a few years prior to the publication of this booklet in the 1960s, the faculty wanted students to give all their attention to nursing and not have any distractions. These students are having their own picnic in the dormitory. (Janelle Adamski.)

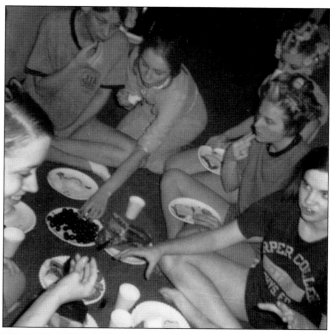

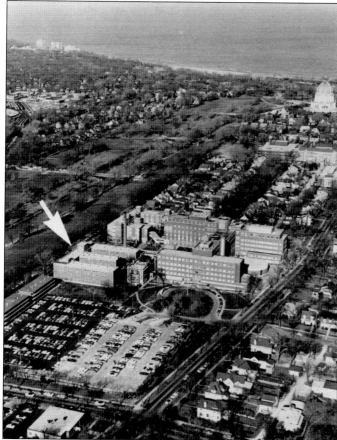

Linda Cranford said of her decision to attend EHSN in 1969, "With Lake Michigan just blocks away and what I thought was an enchanting school, I was sure this was where I wanted to be." (Family of Marjorie Beyers.)

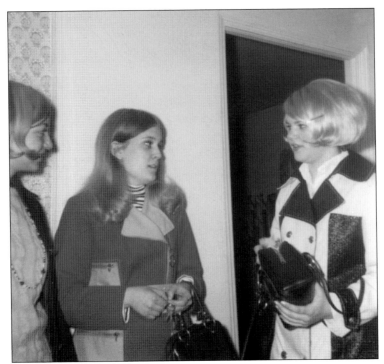

Bikes were available for rent near EHSN, and Roberta Hilliger often rented one, for 15¢, to use as transportation to Baha'i Temple or Lincoln Park Zoo. EHSN had a little sister/big sister program. The big sister was responsible for helping her assigned freshman little sister feel welcomed in the dormitory and at the school. Pictured here are Nancy Bower (center) with her little sister Lisa (left) and classmate Jean Olsen. (Linda Cranford.)

"So You Want to Be a Nurse" mentioned golfing opportunities at the Peter N. Jans Memorial Golf Club (later Canal Shore Golf Club) across the street from the dormitory. Sandra Sill recalls running toilet paper down the fairways for freshman initiation. The course was used more in the evening for student "pinnings" than for daytime golfing. Chad Friedman, a University of Chicago medical student, and Carolyn Smeltzer got pinned on the golf course in 1971. (Carolyn Smeltzer.)

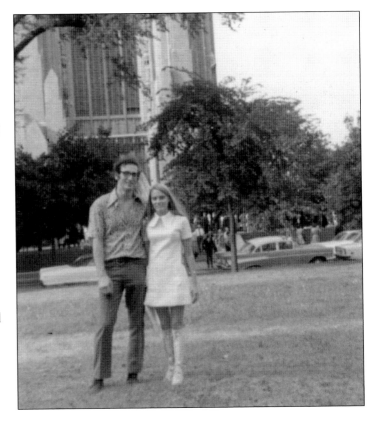

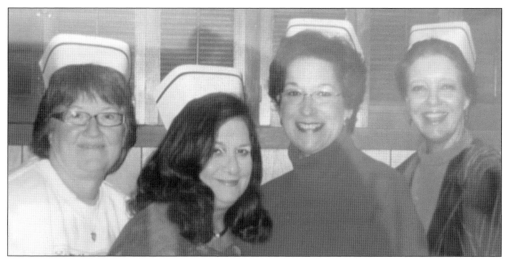

The brochure noted that "attitudes, challenges and opportunities which you will encounter here, and the friendships you will make, will provide enrichment thru-out your life." Kathryn Gray (far right), who started at the school in 1969, stated, "I made lifelong friendships with other women in the dorm." Pictured with Gray from left to right are friends Beth, Deb, and Sue. (Susan Keener.)

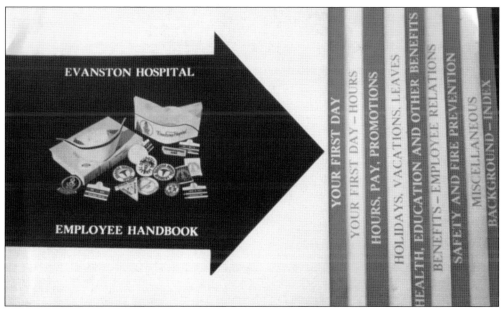

The third section of the brochure, "A Good School," bragged about the accomplishments of EHSN since its inception in 1898. "EHSN has had excellent teaching methods and faculty . . . the school has always gained accreditation, the graduates always placed the highest when taking state boards and the graduates were sought out for employment." Evanston Hospital was always welcoming its own graduates to join its staff, according to Mary Blaisdell. (Barbara McQuillan.)

NURSING SCHO[

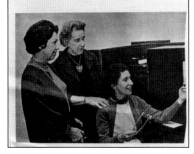

Faculty were always developing new teaching methods and investing in equipment. "So You Want to Be a Nurse" highlighted the low student-to-faculty ratio, which allowed for individual student guidance. Students were treated as staff team members by the hospital's head nurses and nursing staff. There was a great working relationship between the school and the hospital. This article illustrates how the faulty were always seeking out new teaching methods, research, equipment, and tools to enhance the students' learning. (Family of Marjorie Beyers.)

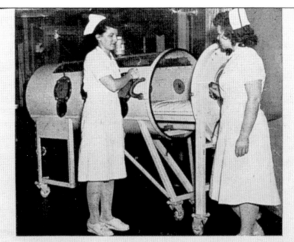

To Help in Our Continuing Fight Against Polio

The respirator above was presented to Evanston Hospital by the Evanston Nurses' Club when that group disbanded in 1947.

Members of the EHSN faculty published many books and articles focusing on refresher tips, case methods of learning, leadership concepts, and critical thinking skills. The faculty created the concept of an open curriculum and published articles on self-paced learning.

Nursing Grad of '28 Publishes Book on Rehabilitation

Mrs. Caroline H. Elledge (Caroline Hubert, class of '28) is the author of a new book, "The Rehabilitation of the Patient," published by J. B. Lippincott Company in June. This small volume, written primarily for laymen, contains many well selected case histories. Mrs. Elledge had excellent opportunity for collecting background for her book while with the Division of Physically Handicapped Children of the New York City Department of Health, and also while a member of the National Council on Rehabilitation. She is now Assistant Professor of social work at McGill University, Montreal.

THE PILOT [15]

The "All Types of Nursing Care" section of "So You Want to Be a Nurse" indicated that EHSN offered experiences with a variety of patients. It highlighted the school's affiliations with other organizations, including the Cradle (an orphanage for babies), the Chicago Maternity Center, and the local nursery school. These experiences offered students an opportunity to care for the healthy child and healthy, pregnant mother.

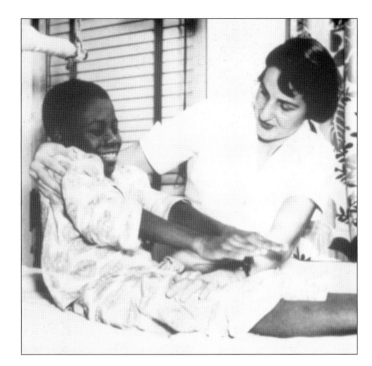

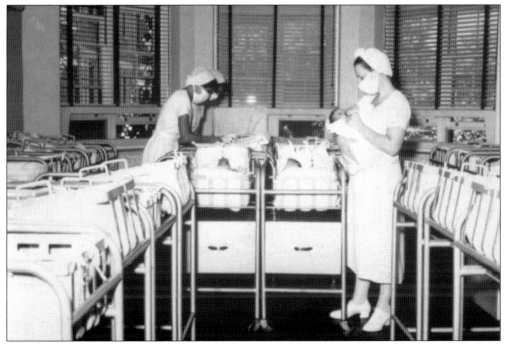

The brochure focused on the fact that training of clinical skills, except for well care and a visiting nurse experience, would be at Evanston Hospital as it was a full-service teaching hospital with many specialties. Before, students went to a variety of hospitals for specific training: Children's Memorial Hospital for pediatrics, Chicago's Lying-in Hospital for maternity, and Cook County Hospital for burns.

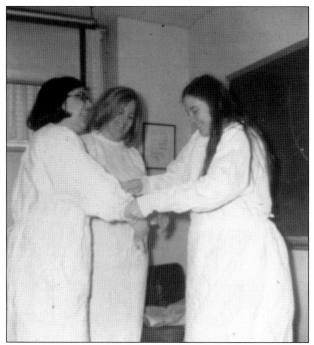

When working with orthopedic patients, students complained that their nursing caps got in the way of the bed's traction bars. The 1972 class asked for and was granted permission to not wear their caps when providing orthopedic care. "We started setting precedents! We paved the way for the future," stated Cheryl Petersen. Pictured here practicing gowning for the operating room are, from left to right, Fran Skafidas, Deborah Nye, and Linda DuBien. (Fran Skafidas.)

EVANSTON HOSPITAL SCHOOL OF NURSING

CLASS OF 1972

1st Quarter
September 8 - November 12, 1969

HOUR	MONDAY	TUESDAY	WEDNESDAY	THURSDAY	FRIDAY
7-8		*week 1-5 9-11*		X-ray Students	
8-9		Nsg.	Nsg. / Integrated Science A_1	Nsg.	Integrated Science *8-9*
9-10	Anatomy & Physiology 9-10:30	A&P Lab 9-11 / Lab 8:30-11	A&P Lab 9-11 / Lab 8:30-11 / Integrated Science A_2	A&P Lab 9-11 / Lab 8:30-11	Anatomy & Physiology 9-10:30
10-11		Gp. A / Gp. B / Integrated Science Gp. C	Gp. B / Gp. C / 9:30-10:30	Gp. C / Gp. A	Integrated Science B_1 10-11
11-12		10-12		Integrated Science Group B_2 11-12	
1-2	Introduction to Nursing	Integrated Science Group A	Integrated Science Group C_1 1-2	Integrated Science C_2 1-2	Introduction to Nursing 1-2
2-3	1-3	1-3		*2 Nursing Math Tests*	Psychology 2-3:30
3-4	Integrated Science 3-4	Integrated Science Group B	Psychology 7-8:30		
4-5		3-5			

"So You Want to Be a Nurse" demonstrated how students would learn skills, science, and nursing fundamentals to care for patients during their freshman year. Fran Skafidas thought the curriculum and faculty were exceptional. After graduation, she attended Marycrest College in Davenport, Iowa. Many of the classes she was required to take there covered material she had already learned at EHSN. (Nancy Miller.)

The brochure emphasized the individual instruction that a student would receive when caring for patients. This picture shows an instructor teaching pediatric care.

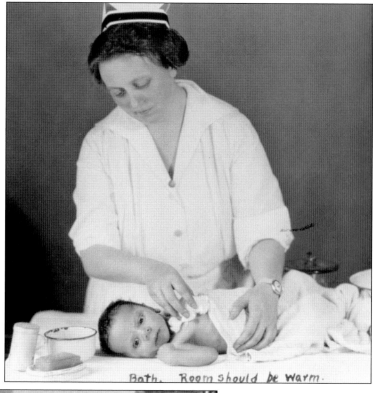

Bath. Room should be warm.

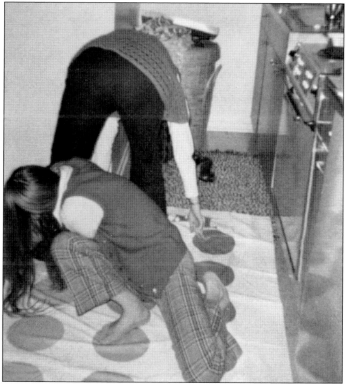

The booklet showed nursing students and faculty interacting. Faculty would hold parties for students that included activities to help them become flexible. The brochure said the ratio of students to faculty was excellent. Between 1969 and 1972 there were 26 faculty and eight administrators, some employed by Northwestern University. The total enrollment was 162, with 40 making up the class of 1972. (Carolyn Smeltzer.)

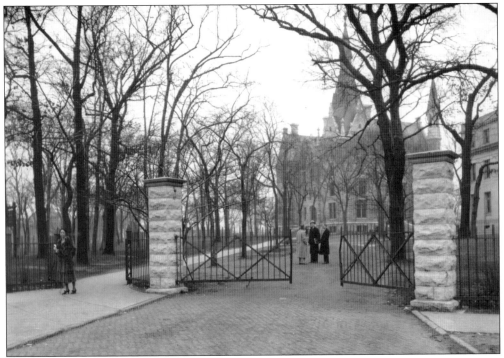

The brochure also mentioned the educational benefits of being associated with Northwestern University, which was within walking distance of Evanston Hospital and the school of nursing. EHSN's relationship with Northwestern dated to 1909. (Archives of Northwestern University.)

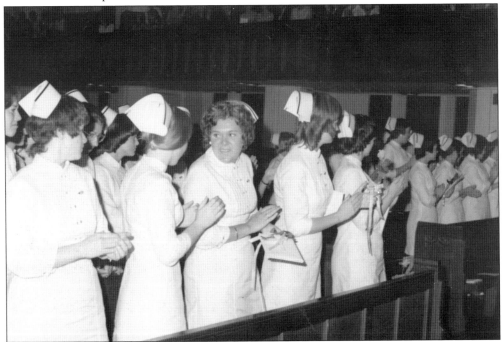

"So You Want to Be a Nurse" romanticized the pinning and graduation ceremonies, with illustrations of joyful students celebrating their accomplishment of becoming a nurse. (Family of Marjorie Beyers.)

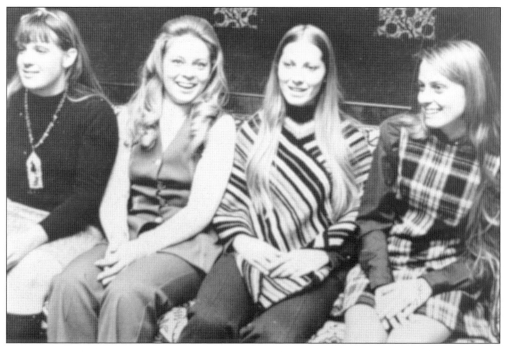

The importance of students gaining skills was highlighted, along with the great living conditions. Students had a private room and beautiful gathering spaces with a kitchenette, shower rooms, bathrooms, and a hall telephone on each floor. EHSN student representatives for the Illinois Student Nurse Association are pictured here. (Carolyn Smeltzer.)

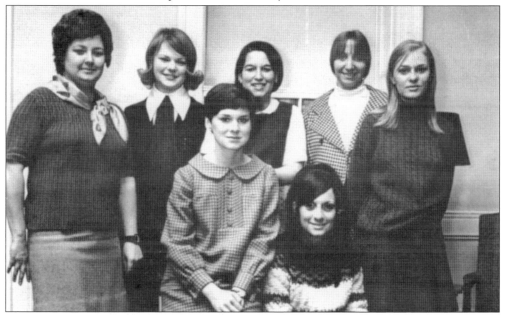

"A Happy and Worthwhile Experience" was the next section of "So You Want to Be a Nurse." It demonstrated that students had many opportunities for leadership or committee involvement, including singing in the chorus or being on the yearbook committee. Members of the class of 1972 are pictured here as freshmen with faculty sponsor Marilyn Keyes (left). (Barbara McQuillan.)

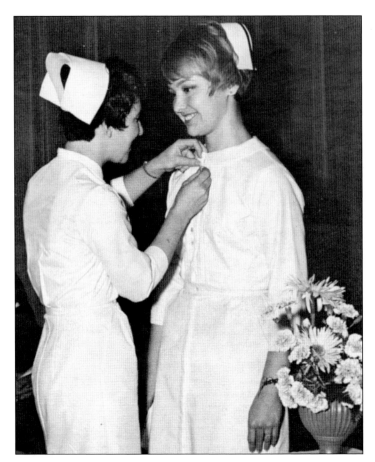

"Career Opportunities" was the final section of the brochure. Opportunities after graduation were outlined along with an urging for students to continue their education. Pictured here is Marjorie Beyers pinning a graduating nurse. (Family of Marjorie Beyers.)

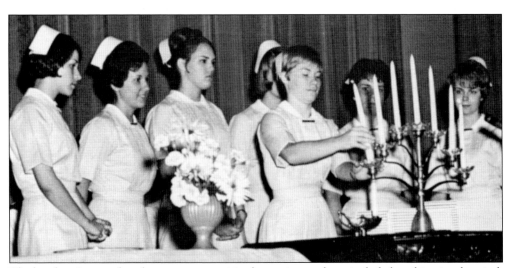

The brochure's examples of career opportunities for nursing students included working in a hospital, at an industrial setting, in a safety and healthcare program, at a business, or joining the armed forces or Peace Corps. Other opportunities included being an airline stewardess or working in a doctor's office. (Family of Marjorie Beyers.)

"So You Want to Be a Nurse" indicated that with more education, nurses could work in public health or at an Indian bureau. It stated that with a college degree, one could advance in administrative or directorial activities, and that the demand for nurses was greater than the supply. A graduate could definitely find a job. Karen Waechter and Linda Cranford both indicated that all the hospitals wanted to hire EHSN graduates because of their excellent training. These images show the front and back of a 1970s Cleveland Clinic recruitment flyer. (Both, Roberta Hilliger.)

NURSING

IS NO BED OF ROSES
amen

... and we're the first to admit it!

Either you or your classmates have met us at conventions. You have at least met us through the mail. Our pamphlets have informed you about the Cleveland Clinic Foundation; our publication, "Under Your Cap", has given you an idea of the quality of patient care as well as the nursing specialties at our hospital; and if you have met with any of us directly, you couldn't help notice the pride we have in being a part of such a world renowned institution.

**Come see for yourself — be our guest
at an open house and get together at the pool!**

For further information regarding the program of the open house, please fill out, detach, and mail the reservation form at your earliest convenience.

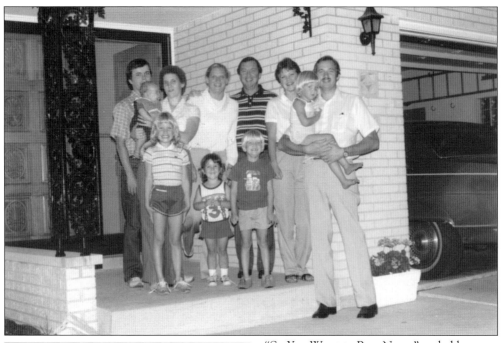

CAP COMMITTEE

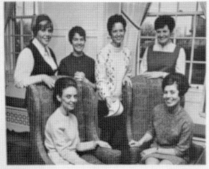

SEATED, LEFT: Mrs Ruth Young, Chairman, Alumni Cap Committee and RIGHT, Mrs. Mary Lynn Ahrens, President, Alumni Association. STANDING LEFT to RIGHT: Maureen Burke, Carolyn Hall, Carole Grennan, Chairman, Student Cap Committee and Mary Beth Schultz. NOT PICTURED: Judy Paige and Kathy Kemmerling.

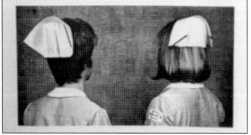

"So You Want to Be a Nurse" ended by stating, "This study of nursing will make you unusually well prepared to be a home maker and mother . . . and the study will help you cope with family illness." Pictured here surrounded by family are three graduates of the class of 1972. From left to right are Marty Grothus Bannon, Linda Cranford, and Nancy Bower Hansen. (Linda Cranford.)

Kathryn Gray said, "EHSN was my first and really only nursing school of choice. . . . I also looked at Oak Park School of Nursing but didn't need any more nuns in my life and was afraid that, like Sally Field, I would fly away in a stiff breeze with that cap!" In 1971, EHSN selected a fourth and final nursing cap with the same back pleat. The previous cap was linen and was retired when the school's cap-cleaner retired. (Barbara McQuillan.)

Roberta Hilliger, president of the class of 1972, said, "I wanted to be a nurse and was attending Northern Illinois University, on the dean's list, but I was bored, bored, bored. I wanted a three-year program associated with Northwestern University. I had never been to Evanston but heard Clark Weber talk about his Evanston adventures on the radio. I transferred to EHSN and lived happily ever after." The Northwestern University campus is pictured here. (Archives of Northwestern University.)

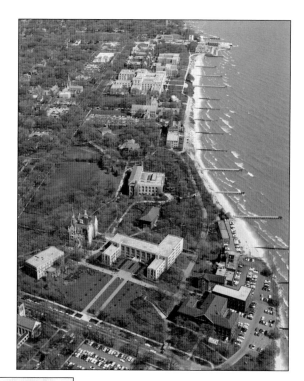

EVANSTON HOSPITAL SCHOOL OF NURSING
2645 GIRARD AVENUE, EVANSTON, ILLINOIS

Dear Miss Schupp,

I am pleased to inform you that the Admissions Committee has reviewed your seventh semester grades and has fully accepted you as a member of the Evanston Hospital School of Nursing class entering in September, 1969.

Will you please confirm your acceptance by sending the matriculation fee of $25.00 by check or money order made payable to the Evanston Hospital Association. In order to reserve your place in the class, this fee should be sent within two weeks of receipt of this letter. Please address your payment to the following:

Mrs. Eleanor Wang, Registrar
Evanston Hospital School of Nursing
2645 Girard Avenue
Evanston, Illinois 60201

At a future date, we will send you information regarding uniform fittings and supplies to bring when you enter in September. If you have questions, however, please feel free to contact me.

Very truly yours,

Virginia Heyer

Virginia Heyer
Admissions Director

VH/sf

Roberta Hilliger said, "I was late transferring to EHSN in the spring. But the girl in the office recognized my voice, and she slipped my paperwork through." Virginia Heyer Nelson, the EHSN admission director, often helped students behind the scenes and signed Nancy Schupp Miller's acceptance letter. (Nancy Schupp Miller.)

Sequence of Nursing Courses		
Nursing	201	Introduction to Nursing
"	202	Medical Nursing
"	203	Surgical Nursing
"	204	Junior Medical Surgical
"	205	Maternity
"	206	Pediatric
"	207	MCH Core Course (Maternal Child Health)
"	208	Senior Integrated Nursing
"	209	Comprehensive
"	210	Psychiatric

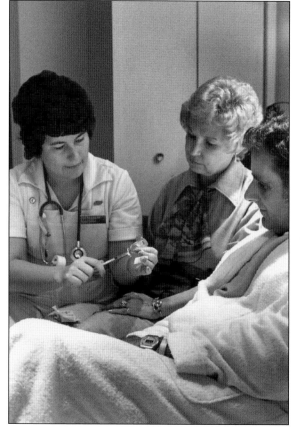

Roseann Boi stated, "I knew my junior year in high school I would attend EHSN or St Francis School of Nursing. I had conversations with a senior friend who chose EHSN, and with a friend's sister who was an EHSN graduate. Both spoke highly of its academic and clinical program. After meeting Marjorie Beyers, the director, and reviewing my research, I decided on EHSN." This image shows a sequence of nursing courses. (Carolyn Smeltzer.)

Barbara McQuillan said, "I was from a small town, and two of my neighbors were EHSN graduates, so I decided that was the school for me. I liked it so much I worked at Evanston Hospital for 48 years." McQuillan is pictured here working as a nurse, teaching the administration of insulin. (Barbara McQuillan.)

Nancy Miller said, "EHSN offered financial aid. This offer of assistance helped me select EHSN, but I never regretted the decision and worked two years at the hospital to repay my loan." This is a typical bill and receipt sent by EHSN after payment was received. The total for this semester in 1971 was $516. (Carolyn Smeltzer.)

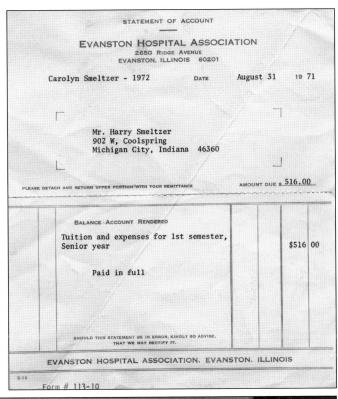

STATEMENT OF ACCOUNT

EVANSTON HOSPITAL ASSOCIATION
2650 RIDGE AVENUE
EVANSTON, ILLINOIS 60201

Carolyn Smeltzer - 1972   DATE   August 31   19 71

Mr. Harry Smeltzer
902 W, Coolspring
Michigan City, Indiana   46360

PLEASE DETACH AND RETURN UPPER PORTION WITH YOUR REMITTANCE   AMOUNT DUE $ 516.00

BALANCE ACCOUNT RENDERED

Tuition and expenses for 1st semester,
Senior year $516 00

Paid in full

SHOULD THIS STATEMENT BE IN ERROR, KINDLY SO ADVISE,
THAT WE MAY RECTIFY IT.

EVANSTON HOSPITAL ASSOCIATION, EVANSTON, ILLINOIS

B-16
Form # 113-10

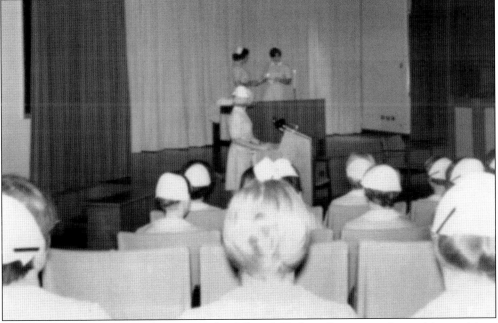

"Evanston was not my first choice," Sandra Sill said. "I chose Evanston after making a visit to the school. The dorm was fantastic, and the curriculum was what I was looking for. It was the right decision for me." Students are pictured during the candle-lighting ceremony for the class of 1972. (Fran Skafidas.)

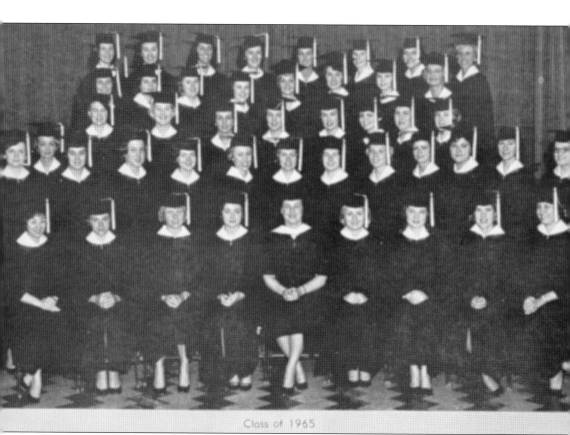

Class of 1965

The class of 1965 is pictured when the group graduated from Northwestern University. After the Northwestern graduation, they had a pinning ceremony at Evanston Hospital.

Four

A Life Worthwhile for You and Me

The Life of a Student Nurse

The first students to attend Evanston Training School for Nurses lived throughout the hospital administration buildings; starting in 1900, students lived in the Cable Building. This residence had a reception area for gathering. From the time the school opened, there was a student library. Students brought washable cotton dresses to wear during their one-month probation period and were later given indoor and outdoor uniforms, along with a non-washable cap to be worn in the hospital and the school. The outdoor uniform was a coat and a hat with a veil.

The early students spent 12 hours on the hospital wards providing patient care and started their class lectures at 8:00 p.m. In 1910, the student's clinical time was reduced to 10 hours per day.

In 1909, the student residence moved to Patten Hall. Ada Belle McCleery, who was then president of the hospital board, stated in her annual report that Patten Hall was the most "complete and beautiful nurses' home in the country." It could house 50 students and had a rooftop garden, kitchen, large library, exercise room, and drawing room. The rules were strict, with little socialization allowed except tea socials. Students could not leave the residence without first reporting to and being granted permission by the nursing superintendent.

Patten Memorial Hall was the nursing residence from 1930 until 1974. Each student had a private room with running water. Each floor had a kitchenette, a community bathroom with showers, and a hall telephone that was manned by switchboard operators. The dormitory had a rooftop where students could sunbathe, a reception hall, a library, science laboratories, an auditorium, and several smaller classrooms.

By 1930, EHSN began hosting Halloween and Christmas parties along with teas and social dances. However, Helen Dulick, class of 1950, said, "There wasn't room for outside activities and interest, nurses should be solely devoted to nursing." This attitude prevailed throughout most of the school's early history.

In the beginning, students had two hours of free time per day for recreation and study along with a half day off on Sundays when possible. Students could not be married and had to live in the school residence. They also obeyed strict bedtime hours, had social limitations, followed rules for behavior, and honored a dress code. The students thrived and became respected nurses.

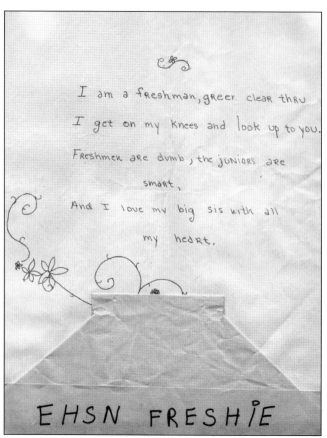

I am a freshman, green clear thru
I get on my knees and look up to you.
Freshmen are dumb, the juniors are smart,
And I love my big sis with all my heart.

EHSN FRESHIE

This chapter is filled with fun pictures that will bring back memories for anyone who lived in a dormitory, especially a nursing dormitory. A student's life involved three main activities: learning, socializing, and spending time providing care in the hospital. Classroom studies included instruction about the art, skill, and science of nursing. (Nancy Miller.)

Students were issued identification cards in order to gain entrance to the hospital. The back of the card contained a description of the student. The information on the back of Carolyn Smeltzer's card included her birthdate, height, weight, hair and eye color, and the statement, "If found, please place in mailbox, postage will be paid." (Carolyn Smeltzer.)

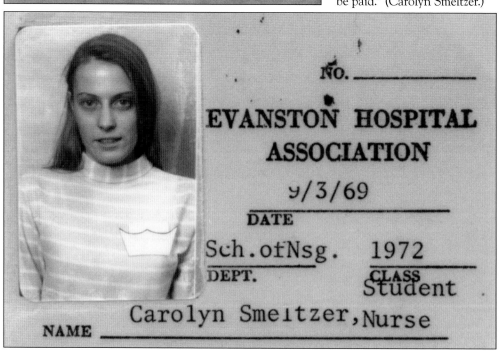

NO. _____

EVANSTON HOSPITAL ASSOCIATION

9/3/69
DATE

Sch. of Nsg.   1972
DEPT.   CLASS
                 Student

Carolyn Smeltzer, Nurse
NAME _____

Life as a student nurse at EHSN focused on learning nursing skills, being a good student, and most importantly, providing care to patients in the hospital. Throughout the years, the goal of the school remained the same—providing education for students to help them become the best possible nurses.

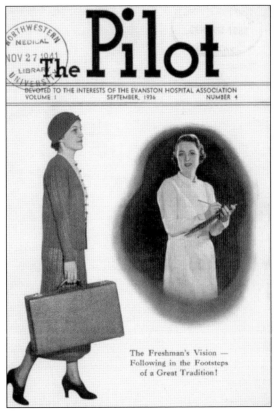

The Freshman's Vision — Following in the Footsteps of a Great Tradition!

In the 1960s, students spent eight hours a day three days a week in the hospital. This left more time for students to socialize and make lifelong friends. Carolyn Smeltzer recalled that celebrations were held "just because—birthdays, Halloween, Christmas, halfway done with school, engagements, Friday nights, start of weekend, good grades, and many more." These students are celebrating at a halfway party. (Nancy Miller.)

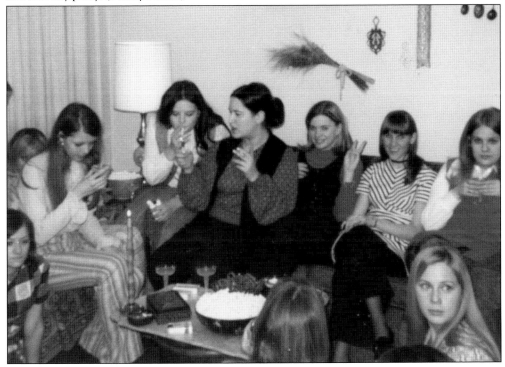

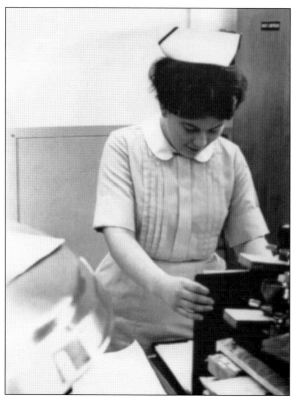

In the 1960s, students received their patient assignments for the following day of clinical in the evening. They then went to the hospital to do patient research and develop a patient care plan. The instructor quizzed the students the following morning on the patients' illnesses, treatment plans, and medications. This student is either charting the progress of her patient or perhaps studying the chart of her next assigned patient. (Barbara McQuillan.).

In their senior year of nursing school, students were in charge of an entire patient care unit. This was a lot of responsibility, but they still had a good time in the dormitory. These students are learning how to take a temperature. (Barbara McQuillan.)

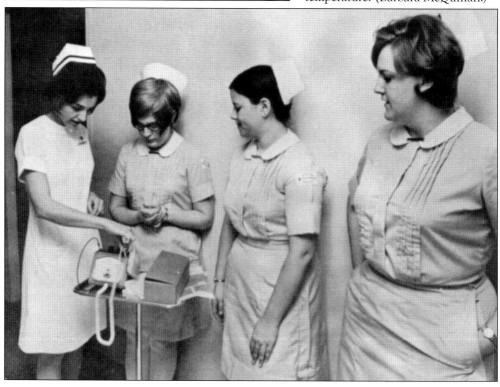

HOUR	MONDAY	TUESDAY	WEDNESDAY	THURSDAY	FRIDAY
8-9		Nurs. Lab Gp. I	Nurs. Lab Gp. I Science Disc. Gp. IIB	Nurs. Lab Gp. II Science Disc. Gp. IA	Nurs. Lab Gp. II
9-10	A&P	Science Lab Gp. II	A&P Lab Gp. II	A&P Lab Gp. I	
10-11	Nursing I & II				
11-12	↓	↓	↓	Science Disc. Gp. IB	↓
12-1	Lunch	↓ Lunch	Lunch	↓	Lunch
1-2	Science Lect.	Science Disc. Gp. IIA	Science 1-2	Lunch	A&P Lect. 1-2
2-3	Science Lab (for ½ students) Gp. I	Nursing I & II	Pharmacology 2-3:30	Nursing I & II	Pharmacology
3-4		↓	↓	↓	↓
4-5	↓				

Throughout their three years of studies, EHSN students had a wide range of experiences caring for all types of patients. The semesters focused on different categories or specialties, such as medical-surgical, pediatrics, maternity, psychiatric, orthopedics, and gastrointestinal disease. This is an example of a freshman's schedule. (Nancy Miller.)

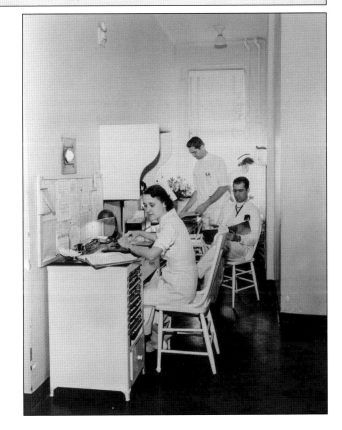

Students were assigned patients who corresponded with what they were studying. The instructors were experts in certain types of illnesses or body functions. The instructors taught the subject and also guided the students on how to care for patients in the hospital. Charting was important for learning and care planning.

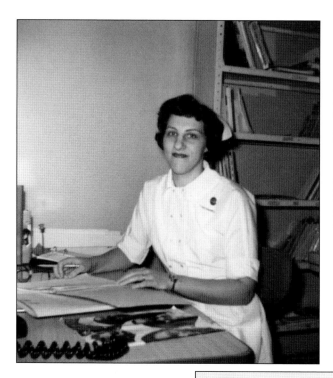

Clinical care is a large part of a nursing student's education. Fran Skafidas stated, "I always admired the professionalism of our instructors. I modeled my own behavior after them. Their knowledge, conduct, and presentation were impressive." Pictured is Dorothy Johnson, instructor of medical-surgical nursing and intensive care nursing and a graduate of Brokaw Hospital School of Nursing and Illinois Wesleyan University. (Family of Marjorie Beyers.)

Marjorie Beyers, who served as the director of EHSN from 1966 to 1980 and taught for one year prior, developed one of the first self-paced learning and testing modules. The modules and exams were created by the instructors. If the student passed the test, she could go on to the next module. This was called an open curriculum. This is an article in the October 1972 *Nursing Outlook* publication written by Beyers and other members of the EHSN faculty. (Barbara McQuillan.)

Mediated Approaches to Learning

Developing a Modular Curriculum

"Redesigned from the inside out" is the authors' description of this revised curriculum that emphasizes auto-tutorial study through the use of a wide range of mediated learning materials.

MARJORIE BEYERS • NANCY DIEKELMANN • MONNA THOMPSON

CHANGE is the idiom of our times. Recognizing this, faculty members at the Evanston Hospital School of Nursing have responded to the changing needs of learners and nursing by redesigning the curriculum from the inside out. Our major purpose was to create an innovative curriculum that would reflect the relevance and futuristic styling demanded in today's world; would meet the varying needs of heterogeneous learners; and would enable both students and teachers to grow professionally.

The authors are all on the faculty of the Evanston Hospital School of Nursing. MISS BEYERS (St. Johns Hospital School of Nursing, Springfield, Ill.; M.S., Indiana University) is director of the school; MRS. DIEKELMANN (B.S.N., Northern Illinois University, DeKalb; M.S. St. Xavier College, Chicago, Ill.) is faculty development coordinator; and MRS. THOMPSON (Evanston Hospital School of Nursing, Ill.; M.S., De Paul University, Chicago, Ill.) is curriculum coordinator.

The change process began in 1964 with assessment of the strengths and weaknesses in the existing curriculum. Among the strengths were well-defined content, as a result of previous curriculum revisions, and instructors who were competent nurses in specialized areas of practice. Major weaknesses were that (1) slow and rapid learners were, in effect, penalized by academic routines designed for "average" students; and (2) content taught in class was often not directly related to clinical practice experiences. We knew that students retained content better when it was directly applied to patient care but, because the content followed a prescribed sequence, there were not enough patients with the specific problems being discussed in class to give every student the appropriate experience. Thus, students had to study different content for lecture and for clinical practice.

We therefore decided to examine the relationships among content units. The content in the existing curriculum followed a simple to complex order and/or an order perceived by the teacher as a natural progression. So, as a beginning, we decided that within any given course students could study content in any sequence. This meant that different students could study different units of content at the same time, thus enabling faculty to plan more relevant patient care experiences and to better integrate content and its clinical application.

Before initiating this new system, however, we had to analyze our philosophy of teaching and learning. We asked ourselves:
1. How could different students study different content areas at the same time?
2. Could a flexible order of content arrangement be valid in terms of prerequisites and content complexity?
3. Would the flexible order lessen the value of students' sharing content in seminar groups?
4. How would the flexible order affect evaluation techniques?
5. What controls would be neces-

OCTOBER, 1972 VOL. 20, NO. 10

643

EHSN instructors had to have a bachelor's degree. Some of the faculty members, if not most, were only a few years older than the students. The instructors were recruited from all over the country. Many of them wrote books and articles. Some were national speakers and influencers on the art and science of nursing. Marjorie Beyers received her doctorate from Northwestern University; she is pictured here as a graduate nurse. (Family of Marjorie Beyers.)

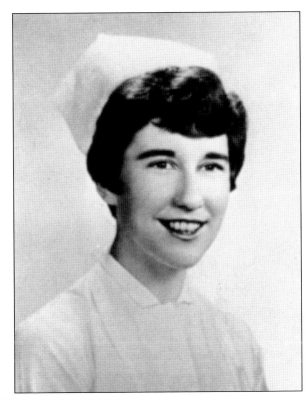

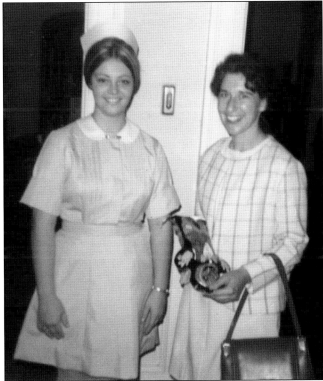

Marjorie Beyers grew up on a farm in southern Illinois and never forgot her roots. She was known as Aunt Margie to her nephews and nieces. To EHSN graduates and faculty, she was known as a mentor with visionary and creative thinking skills who made an impact on their lives. Dr. Beyers graduated from the University of Indiana and St. John's College of Nursing. She is pictured here (at right) with an unidentified EHSN student nurse. (Family of Marjorie Beyers.)

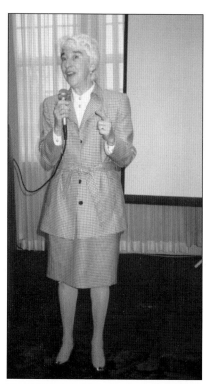

Marjorie Beyers held many leadership roles, serving as executive director of the National Commission on Nursing, vice president of nursing and allied health at Mercy Health Services, director of the American Organization of Nursing Executives, and as a tenured professor at the University of Texas. During her retirement, she was the interim chancellor at St. John's College in Springfield, Illinois, and a member of numerous national healthcare boards. (Family of Marjorie Beyers.)

Marjorie Beyers wrote several books, including *Leadership in Nursing Management*, *The Clinical Practice of Medical-Surgical Nursing*, *Nursing Management for Patient Care*, *Complete Guide to Cancer Nursing*, and numerous articles. She taught nursing leadership at EHSN to the class of 1972 from the rough draft of her book *Leadership in Nursing Management*. Marjorie Beyers died in 2022—the year of the 1972 class's 50th reunion, where she was honored. (Family of Marjorie Beyers.)

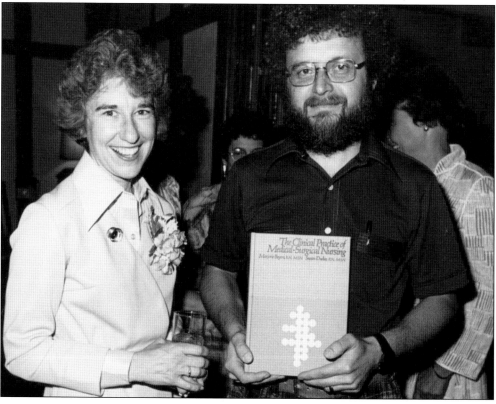

On the night of January 8, 1972, a fire occurred in the dormitory's library. The students were awakened by the alarm in each room. They left their rooms and went down the stairwell to get outside. Eventually, all students were given a bed in the hospital. No one was injured. Pictured is Linda Cranford's room, which was typical, but neater than most. Note the cap hanging from the lamp shade, which kept it firm, in shape, and clean. (Linda Cranford.)

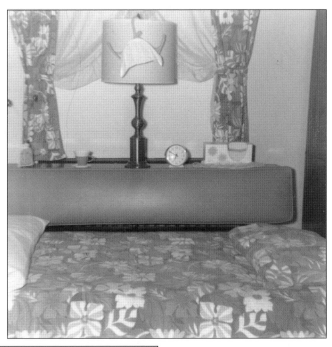

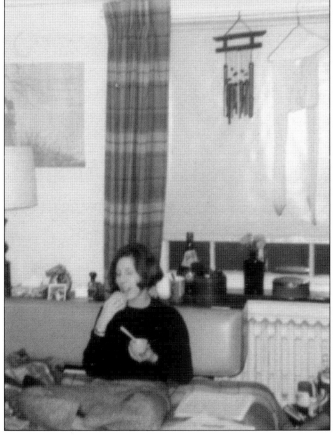

Sandra Sill (pictured) recalls, "I remember the morning I turned on Girard and saw all the fire trucks and police cars outside Patten Memorial Hall, hoping all my classmates were okay. The library was gone, but everyone got out all right. I had just gotten married in December, so was living off campus. It was a terrible sight not knowing what had happened to all my friends and those living in the dormitory." (Carolyn Smeltzer.)

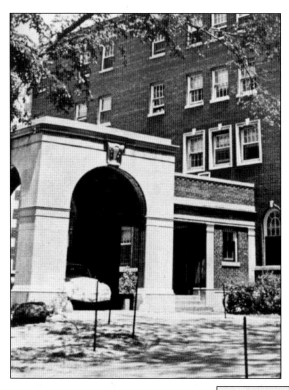

All of the students' parents were personally called about the school fire. Parents were notified that there were no injuries and that the students would have to return home for a week. A newspaper article stated that there was $65,000 of damage. Patten Memorial Hall is pictured here.

This article about the fire stated that Monna Thompson, a faculty member, was the coordinator who directed the cleanup after the fire and reorganized the curriculum. (Barbara McQuillan.)

Fire Destroys School of Nursing Audio-Visual Area on Jan. 6

166 Students Evacuate Safely
Damage Estimated At $65,000

A fire of major proportions destroyed the audio-visual center in the school of nursing on January 6. A preliminary investigation determined that the cause was electrical in nature, resulting in an estimated $65,000 in damage. The fire seemed to have originated in the audio-visual area, which was filled with 20 carrels, equipped with slide projectors and recorders. The alarm sounded at 5:04 A.M. The heat and smoke from the A.V. room extended into the nursing arts lab in which three TV monitors and three video tape recorders were burned, according to Miss **Monna Thompson**, Curriculum Coordinator, who directed the reorganization and clean-up. The Learning Resource Center reading room was damaged by smoke and water. The 166 students living in the dormitory were safely evacuated to the hospital cafeteria and were able to return to their rooms, which took only minor smoke. For the past 1½ yrs. the school has been developing a project in which all teaching materials had been transferred over to audio-visual aids as part of a self-paced curriculum, which served as the bulk of the teach-

ing program along with conferences and seminars. Approximately a year ago the media room in the learning center was completely remodeled from an old amphitheater-type classroom, carpeted throughout. Classes began again on January 10, after a one-day clean-up by faculty and students who removed and washed books on January 7. Faculty and students are attempting to carry on the flexible open curriculum with the remaining resources. The chemistry lab is being used as a tem-

porary library and adjoining microbiology lab is being used for a reading room. About 20 percent of the slides and 50 percent of the audio tapes were recovered. The video tapes and movies are still being evaluated. "Plans are underway for the reconstruction of a new media room and for rennovation of the media. The learning resource center will be operating, on a limited basis, in temporary quarters, soon," said Miss **Marjorie Beyers**, Director of the school.

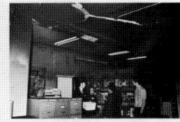

Mr. Ken Sergent, Administrative Resident; Miss Thompson, Mr. Rouse, Controller, and Wayne Hanley, Engineering, discuss the damage.

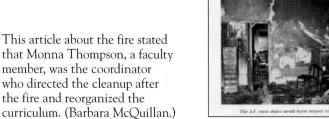

The A.V. room shows carrels burnt beyond rerogation.

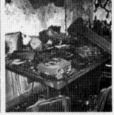

A steel beam rests on the table which holds two charred carousels.

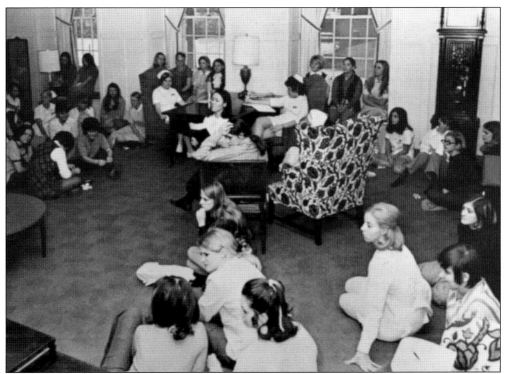

Marjorie Beyers held a student meeting in Patten Memorial Hall regarding the fire and said, "The library modules for learning were destroyed in the fire, instructors have to organize their lectures, and you, the students, should go home for a week's vacation." This message was delivered with a positive attitude and a smile on her face. (Barbara McQuillan)

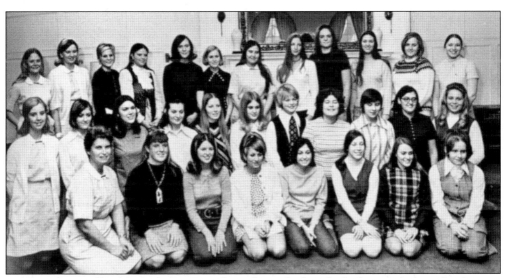

Carol Beebe recalls "during the winter, taking the path though the basement from the dorm to the hospital for clinicals in order to stay warm" and "signing in and out of the front desk when leaving the campus." The EHSN class of 1972 is pictured here during the group's junior year. (Barbara McQuillan.)

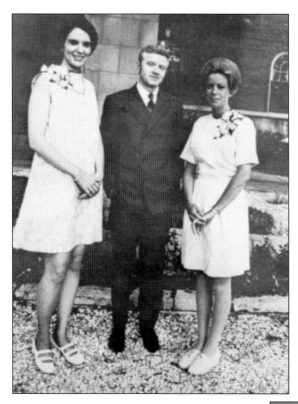

The instructors at EHSN were remarkable, young, and energetic. They mingled with students, participated in skits, and hosted parties. Each year, the class voted to choose their teacher of the year. The 1972 freshman class chose Dr. Reid James, a Northwestern University faculty member who taught anatomy and physiology. Their junior year, they chose Marilyn Keyes. Pictured here from left to right are Nancy Orth, psychiatric nursing instructor; Dr. James; and Marion "Missy" (Kahn) Rodey, nutrition instructor. (Carolyn Smeltzer.)

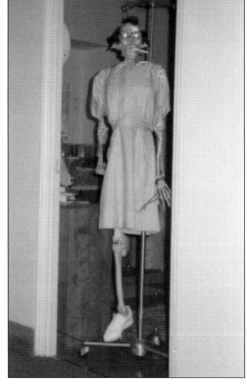

Dr. Reid James made learning fun as well as challenging. Every day of class, he would pull from a container a name of a student and ask a question about their assignment. The correctness of the answer would be woven into the student's final grade. Outside of Dr. James's office was a skeleton (pictured here in 1970), which sometimes got dressed up as a student by the students. (Janelle Adamski.)

Dr. Reid James also taught the muscles of the body by showing a *Playboy* centerfold on the big-screen projector. His final test asked students to identity the muscles in a dissected rat, while he gave this advice: "Don't stand still and passively watch the world go by, because if you do . . . it will." The students took his words to heart, always celebrating birthdays with a toilet-papered room and cake. Pictured is Fran (Vretis) Skafidas's birthday party. (Carolyn Smeltzer.)

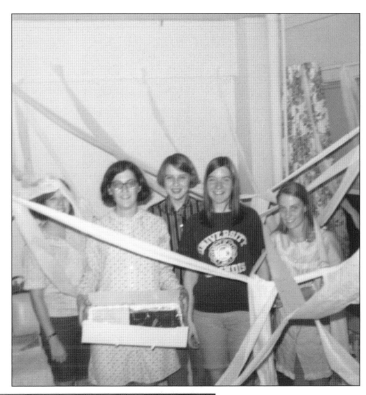

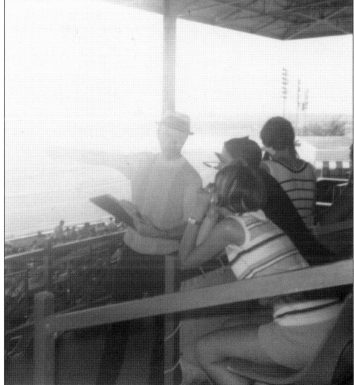

As freshmen, the members of the class of 1972 were invited to the race track by Dr. James. He said he wanted students to compare a horse's body to a human body. In reality, he was rewarding the class at the end of their freshman year, as all the students had achieved a B or higher in anatomy and physiology. (Linda Cranford.)

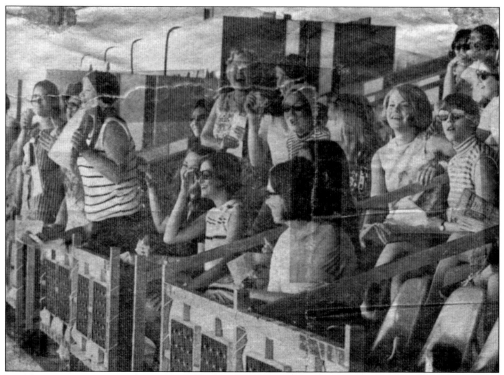

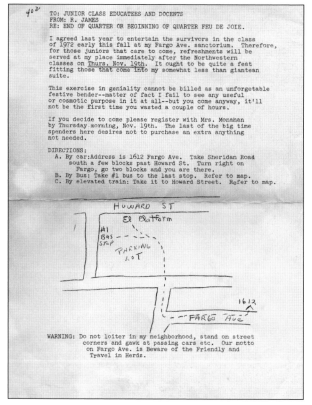

This photograph appeared in the June 14, 1970, *Chicago Sun-Times* featuring the students at the Arlington race track. The caption read, "Student nurses from Evanston Hospital School of Nursing visit Arlington Park for a day at the races. From their expressions, it looks like some of them came up with some winners." (Nancy Miller.)

Dr. Reid James, whom many called Dr. Reid, said, "With being on the hospital premises, your on-site learning experiences were superior to those programs where students were exposed to real hospital situations in more limited ways." Cheryl Petersen recalls Dr. James going to his office one day to find it covered with toilet paper. The next day, after his office was filled with balloons, he changed the locks on his door. (Nancy Miller.)

Dr. Reid James also said, "Since you lived together right at the hospital, you were able to establish meaningful relationships with each other and your nursing instructors." Fifty years ago, he gave this advice to the students: "I encourage you to adopt an expansive philosophy and not be consumed by conflict. In this little chapter of your life, you have toiled." Students are pictured celebrating their last anatomy and physiology exam with his skeleton. (Janelle Adamski.)

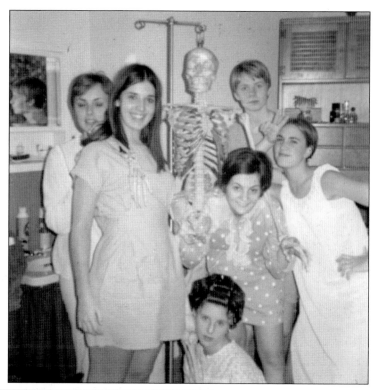

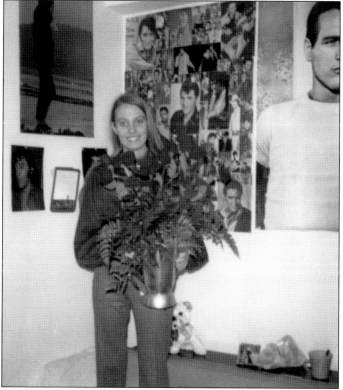

Today, 50 years later, Dr. James said, "I remember most how we supported each other as faculty and students. We knew what the common goal was . . . to launch as far as possible the greatest number of students on a successful career." Carolyn Smeltzer recalls that the biggest debate amongst students was who was the most talented—Elvis Presley, the Beatles, or Tom Jones. Roberta Hilliger, the class president, skipped graduation dinner to attend an Elvis concert. (Carolyn Smeltzer.).

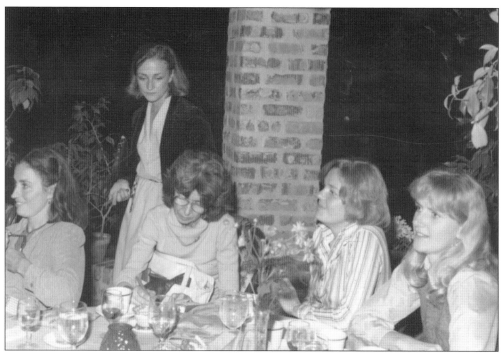

Other instructors included Monna Thompson, an EHSN graduate with degrees from the University of Illinois and DePaul; Alma Labunski, a diploma graduate with a degree from Wheaton College; Sheila Haas; and Ruth Young, another EHSN graduate with a degree from Northwestern University. Pictured here are Merry Ann Hellrung Pearson (far left) and Norma Tribble Hoaglund (far right), both medical-surgical instructors. (Family of Marjorie Beyers.)

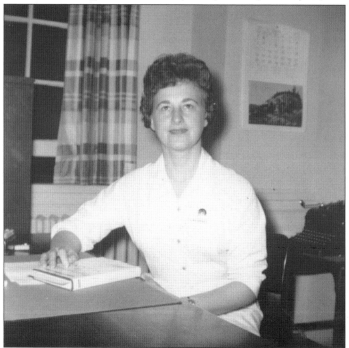

Dorothy Johnson Danielson (pictured) served as a faculty member and director of the school, and in 1966, she was chairperson of the department of nursing. She was a founder of the American Organization of Nurse Executives. Dr. Sheila Haas became dean of Loyola School of Nursing and Dr. Alma Labunski became the dean of North Park. Norma Hoaglund became the vice president for nursing at Glenbrook Hospital. (Family of Marjorie Beyers.)

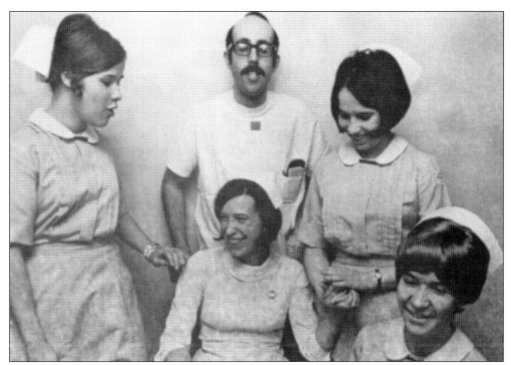

Instructor Suzanne O'Connell (seated at center) married a Smeltzer. Her husband and one of her students had the same last name, and both had family in Pennsylvania. By the 1980s, the nursing community had two Dr. Smeltzers with EHSN roots. Suzanne, a retired Villanova University professor, and Carolyn, a retired PricewaterhouseCoopers partner, recently wrote books. Suzanne wrote *Delivering Quality Healthcare for People with Disabilities*, and Carolyn is one of the authors of this book. Suzanne is pictured with students. (Barbara McQuillan.)

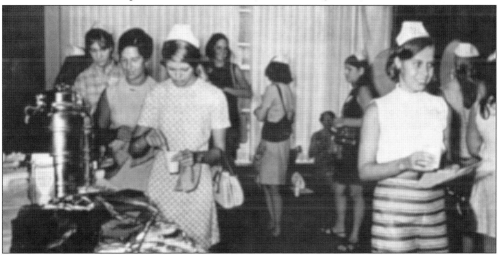

Missy Rodey, the nutritional instructor, stated, "I loved watching young women come in as freshmen with their nervous anticipation and grow through the years into confident, skilled nurses. I admired their choice of a career and dedication to classes and patients . . . students made me a better teacher. . . . Students said one test was too hard and unfair, so I threw it out." (Barbara McQuillan.)

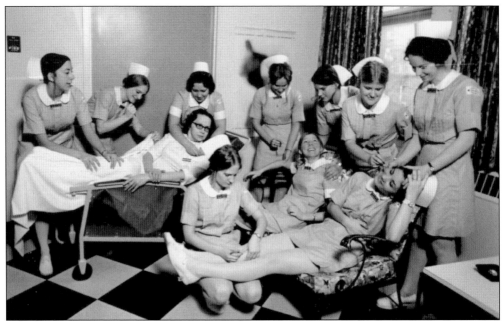

Medical-surgical instructor Marilyn Leczinski Carpenter said, "I remember so many wonderful times. The students were delightful, funny, and very smart. The faculty got along so well, and many of us became lifelong friends. What a blessing experience in my life! I remember skit night and the talent show. At one, there was a meringue pie to the face of a faculty member that did not go well as a joke." Carpenter continued, "After a clinical portion of the day, the student and I talked and shared our concerns about a patient. The next day, the same student and I walked in his room, his bed was stripped, and we looked at each other and asked where was he transferred to; of course, he had died." The students studied theory and did clinical skill practice on mannequins and other students, but mostly on patients. (Below, Fran Skafidas.)

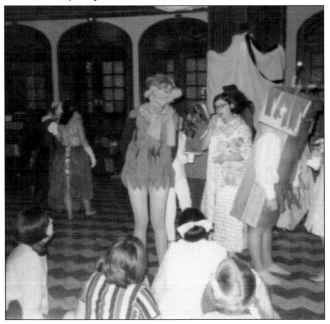

Marilyn Leczinski Carpenter said, "One day, there was an order for antibiotic eye drops and antibiotic ointment for a different part of the body. Yep! the student put the topical ointment in the patient's eye, an incident report was filled out, and the patient survived!" Pictured here are Louise Scalbom (left), director of EHSN student health, and Viola Shimkus, EHSN secretary. (Family of Marjorie Beyers.)

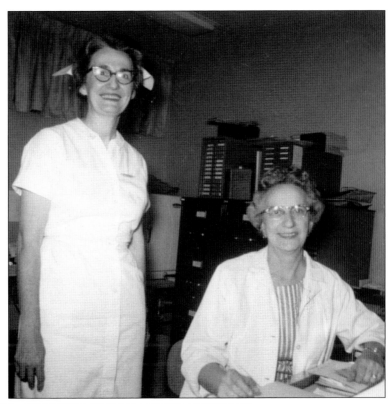

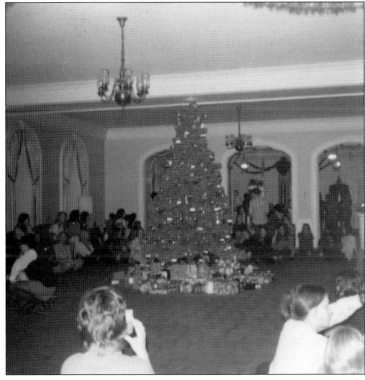

Marilyn Leczinski Carpenter went back to Patten Memorial Hall prior to it being demolished and stated, "It was an eerie experience. Parts of the building looked familiar . . . and parts totally unrecognizable; I was so sad, I couldn't locate my office, nor Marilyn Keyes's office, which was at the end of the hall with all the pencils and papers neatly on the desk." Patten Memorial Hall is shown during Christmas. (Nancy Miller.)

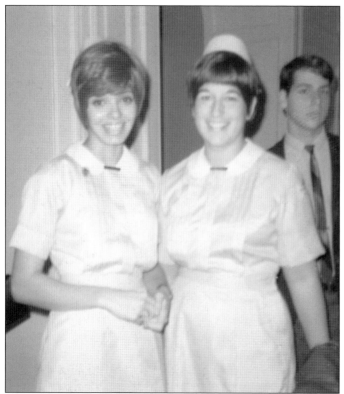

The EHSN faculty created the learning environment and shaped the students' lives. The instructors were unique, as most of them became national nursing leaders. Susan Keener, a member of the class of 1972, said, "I have told people that my education instilled a problem-solving process regardless of the endeavors I undertook." Pictured here are Kathryn Gray (left) and Susan Keener. (Janelle Adamski.)

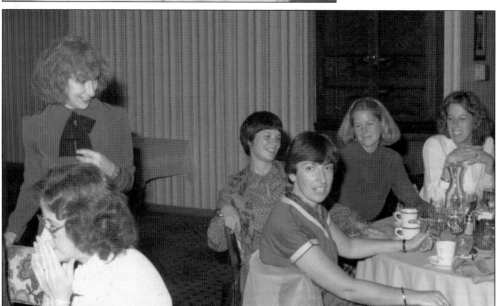

Carolyn Smeltzer was fortunate to work and maintain relationships with several faculty members after graduation. She worked at Loyola University with Shelia Haas and was a consultant with Merry Ann Pearson. Smeltzer continued creatively thinking with Marjorie Beyers (standing at left) throughout her nursing career. Sheila Haas, a medical-surgical instructor, faces the camera at center. (Family of Marjorie Beyers.)

The members of the class of 1972 remember Robert Redford once picking up his nurse date at Patten Memorial Hall. Since the switchboard was manned at times by students, all of them knew when he was arriving. Students gathered to see one of the stars of *Butch Cassidy and the Sundance Kid*, which was showing down the street from the dormitory on Central Avenue. No secrets were left untold in the dormitory. (Carolyn Smeltzer.)

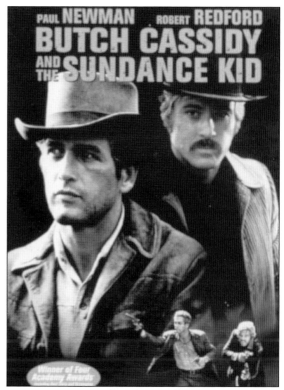

Robert Redford picked up his date and escorted her to the Playboy Club in Lake Geneva, Wisconsin. It certainly made the Friday night exciting for the students. One student walked up to him and said, "If you are Robert Redford, I am Elizabeth Taylor." This was recalled by Roberta Hilliger, a student switchboard operator, who was amazed at how short Redford was. (Carolyn Smeltzer.)

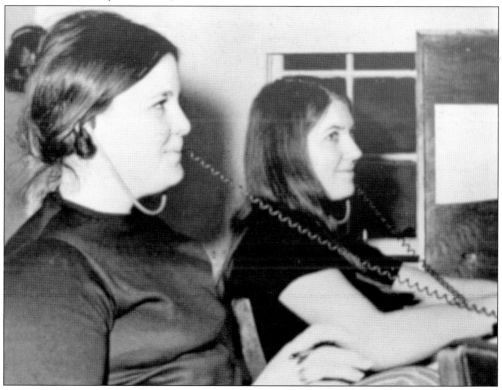

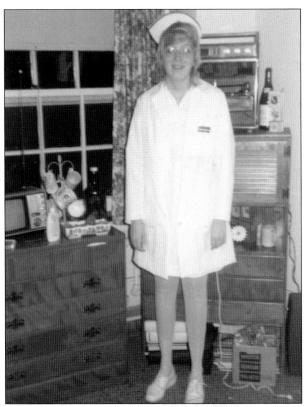

Students' cleaning chores included the dormitory halls and the refrigerator in the kitchenette. According to Katherine Carroll (pictured), "We kept our milk on the window shelves in our room for coldness and safekeeping. The students were reluctant to throw out spoiled food that stunk but not as reluctant to help themselves to the 'good food' when hungry. The owners of the missing food would then make a stink." According to Carroll, "The taking of 'good' food when hungry did not seem to be an issue. Students yelled, 'What happened to my food, it's gone!' " For Carolyn Smeltzer's 20th birthday, she was given a package of steaks by her classmate Juliette Robinson. Fifty-one years later, Carolyn still does not know which student(s) had a nice dinner with her birthday steaks. Beth Ann Baker is pictured below. (Left, Katherine Carroll; below, Janelle Adamski.)

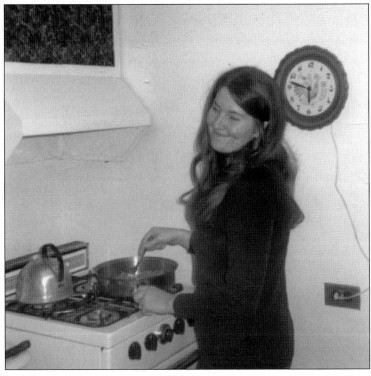

Roberta Hilliger made a tie-dyed granny dress out of the clean yellow sheets the students were issued every Tuesday. Mrs. Cromwell, the "laundress spokesperson," saw Hilliger wearing the fashionable dress around the dormitory. On the next sheet exchange day, Mrs. Cromwell told Hilliger she was no longer in the sheet-exchange program. This is a yellow pillowcase made from the same fabric as that sheet 50 years later. (Linda Cranford).

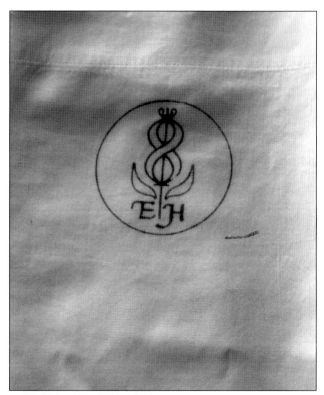

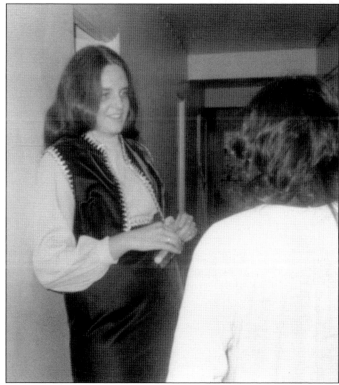

At the end of the year, with a twinkle in her eye, Mrs. Cromwell asked Roberta Hilliger to make a tie-dyed sheet dress for her. Hilliger, 1972 class president and graduation speaker, is pictured here. (Nancy Miller.)

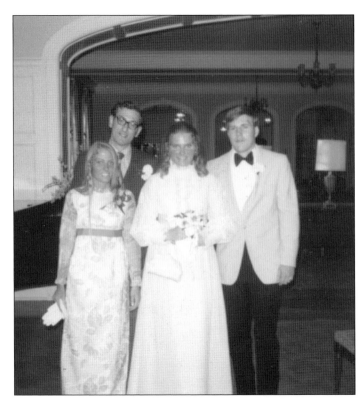

Linda Cranford recalled a memory of Patten Memorial Hall after curfew as "a large room with a couple of recessed sitting rooms, the grand piano, and the Queen Anne chairs. I can never forget sneaking past the guard that sat just left of the entrance door to get to the elevator or stairs when we were past curfew—and *oh*, that elevator!" Pictured in Patten Memorial Hall before a formal dance are, from left to right, Carolyn, Chad, Linda, and Dan. (Carolyn Smeltzer)

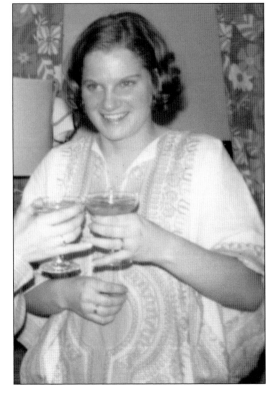

Linda Cranford said, "I do remember the buzzer in each room that, when pushed, alerted us to an all-assemble in the gym for an announcement of an engagement. This occurred usually in the evening or at night, so we all were in our pajamas! Then there was one night when the vending machine went wacko, and we got free candy." Cranford is pictured celebrating her short-term engagement. (Carolyn Smeltzer.)

According to Linda Cranford, "I remember my classmates made me a Mother Goose Award because I had given the most enemas during a rotation. Seems a doctor had inquired about me, as no patient of mine ever had to be rescheduled due to incomplete prep." There was always a big gathering at the mailboxes on the first floor of Patten Memorial Hall. All mail was welcomed—except a notice about rat duty. All 1972 EHSN graduates had to perform rat duty, which consisted of feeding the laboratory rats and cleaning their cages. Late in the school year, the rats were gassed, and the class dissected them as part of their final exam. Mary Blaisdell once got a note from the switchboard operator telling her of her upcoming "rat duty," and she kept the note (below) for over 53 years. (Right, Carolyn Smeltzer; below, Mary Blaisdell.)

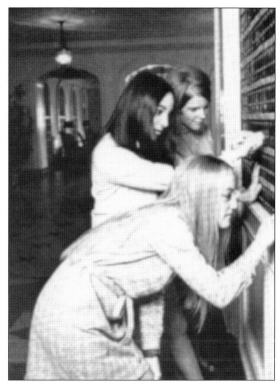

Form B-41

EVANSTON HOSPITAL ASSOCIATION
Telephone Message

For: Miss Callahan

From: Mr. James

Telephone No:

You are scheduled for rat duty on Wed. of this week

Date:

Time:

Receiver:

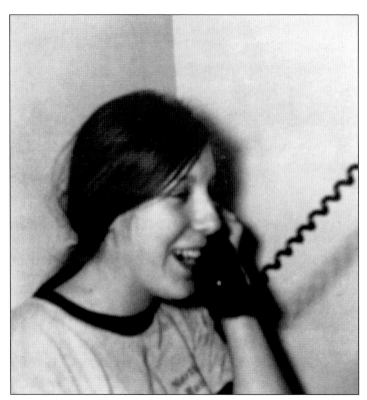

Each hall had a telephone, and students had a limit on how long they could talk, as other students were always awaiting important calls. Roberta Hilliger said, "One student put a bottlecap on her buzzer so she would know if she missed a phone call when she was out of her room." Sandra Sill is pictured on the community hall telephone. (Carolyn Smeltzer)

According to Roberta Hilliger, "In October of 1971, my then-boyfriend David, a conscientious objector working at the hospital, asked if I wanted to go with him to learn transcendental meditation at the Alice Millar Chapel on Northwestern University's campus . . . I did, and now it's been over 50 years that I've been meditating." Many students brought their parents to see Hilliger's room, since it was always decorated in hippie style with beads. (Carolyn Smeltzer.)

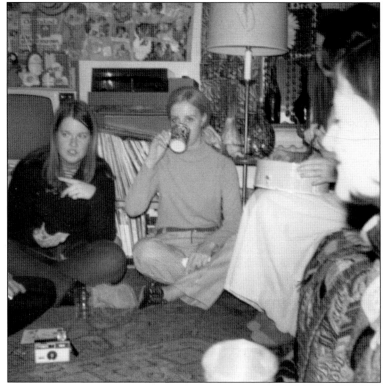

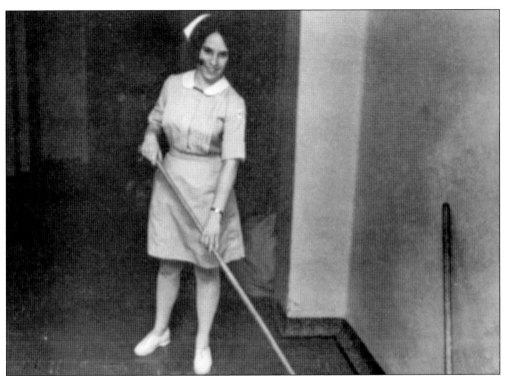

Kathryn Gray recalls mopping the floors, cleaning the kitchens, making Rice-a-Roni dinners in the popcorn-maker, eating deep-dish pizza at Inferno's, and stopping for hot dogs at Mustards Last Stand. Such was the life of a student. Roseann Boi is shown cleaning the halls in her uniform. (Barbara McQuillan.)

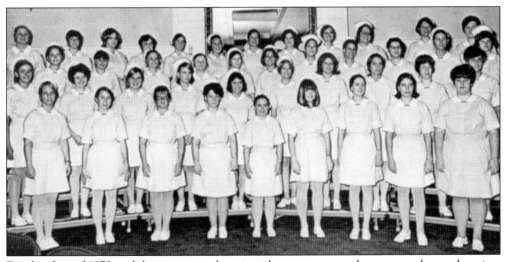

For the class of 1972, it did not matter what time they went out—what mattered was what time they came in. Friday and Saturday nights had a curfew of 10:00 p.m., while all other nights had a curfew of 9:00 p.m. unless a student's parents gave them permission to stay out later when babysitting or singing at a concert. If a student was late and got caught, she had to present to the faculty committee about why she was late. (Carolyn Smeltzer.)

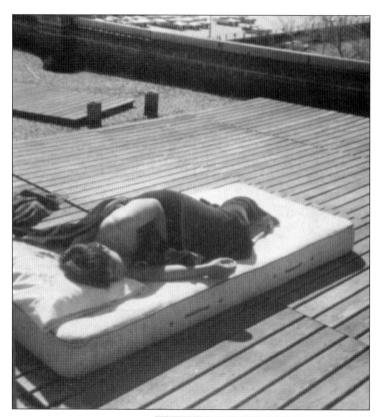

Students would go to the rooftop in the spring with baby oil covering their bodies, lay on a tinfoil mat, and bask in the sun. Sometimes, they would even take their nursing books to study. Sunning on the rooftop was actually promoted as a benefit of choosing EHSN as a place of study. (Barbara McQuillan.)

One night, Roberta Hilliger decided to camp on the rooftop , not realizing security would lock the door. She had to wait until morning to identify De Ann's window; she knocked and woke her up and asked, "Will you open the rooftop door so I will not be late for clinical?" These students are standing in a dormitory room—note the sink in the room. All EHSN dormitory rooms had running water. The school advertised this feature in its brochure for prospective students. (Barbara McQuillan.)

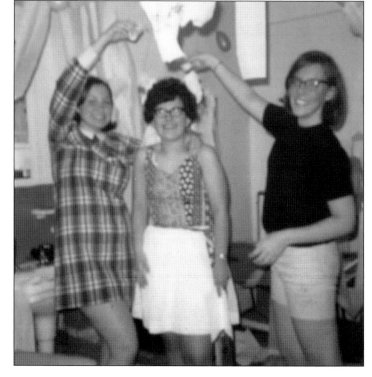

104

Men were only allowed to visit in a dormitory room on Sunday afternoon with parental permission. Moving day was an exception, as fathers could help load and unload students' belongings. When a man was spotted on the floor, students would yell, "man on floor" to alert other students so they would be properly dressed. (Barbara McQuillan.)

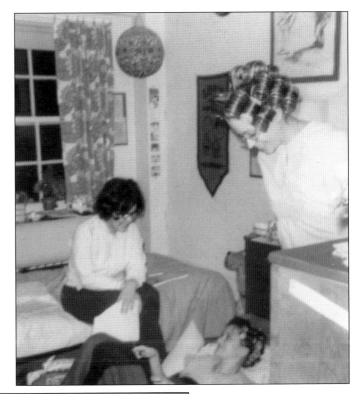

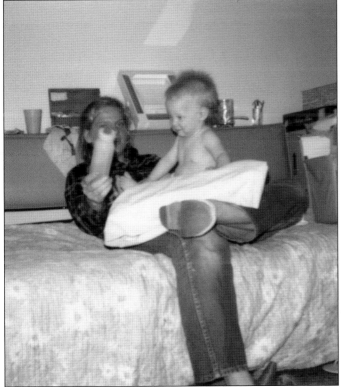

For their maternity rotation, students were assigned a "mother to be." They followed the mother through pregnancy and were on call for her delivery. Cheryl Petersen's assigned mother delivered a baby boy the day before Petersen's birthday. While working in maternity, the students often picked up babysitting jobs. Linda Cranford is shown babysitting Mathew DuBien while his mother was in class; Mathew was the only male visitor who was allowed into the dormitory at any time. (Carolyn Smeltzer.)

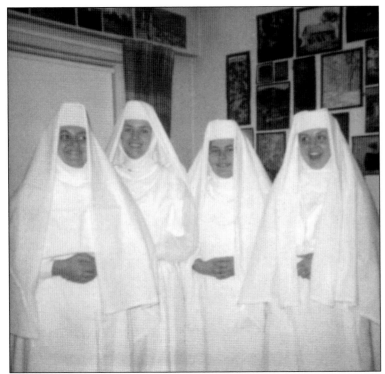

The Halloween party was a big occasion at EHSN, and the tradition dated to the early 1900s. Faculty and students joined in the fun by dressing up in costumes. All of them enjoyed each other's creativity. These student nurses transformed into nuns in habits. (Fran Skafidas.)

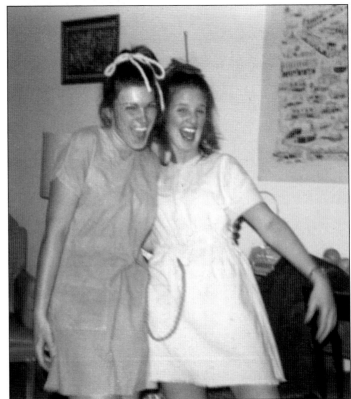

The student nurses put a lot of effort and creativity into their Halloween outfits. This pair of "twins" is connected by an umbilical cord. (Janelle Adamski.)

106

These freshman students got in the spirit of Halloween. It was not the only party they grooved to, as Friday nights in the dormitory often led to some sort of party or fun activity. Because students had no responsibilities for the weekend except studying and perhaps a babysitting job, Friday nights were special. (Janelle Adamski.)

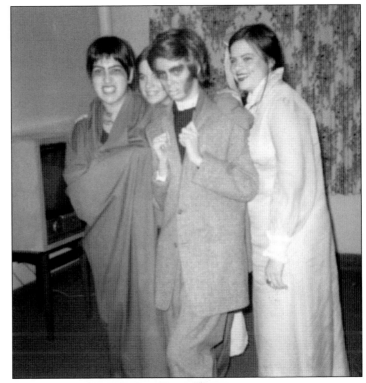

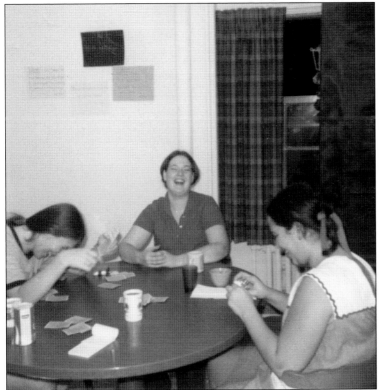

Staying in on a Friday night was not boring. Students played cards and games, listened to music, made dinners, danced, rehashed the week, and sometimes talked about faculty. Cheryl Petersen can still remember Cynthia Dunsmore, the maternity instructor, and her favorite phrase, "Suffice it to say," and the guidance counselor, Kathryn Beadle, having a little car that sounded like a lawnmower. (Nancy Miller.)

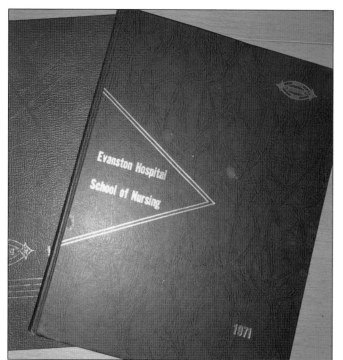

The students recorded their fun and study with an annual yearbook. The first yearbooks of EHSN were called the *Lens*, the next were named *Patterns* (of student life), and later, the yearbooks had no names. These later books only had a symbol of the nursing pin on top of the cover and the year of publication on the bottom. (Rebecca Hilliger and Katherine Carroll.)

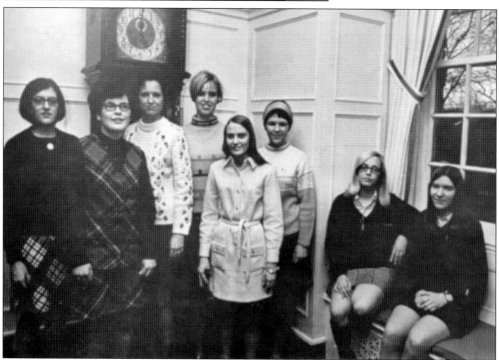

The *Lens* had formal pictures trimmed in a fancy frame, in contrast to the later yearbooks that displayed pictures in a much more casual manner to mirror the freer style of life in the dormitory. The last EHSN yearbook was printed in 1971. A yearbook committee is pictured here. (Carolyn Smeltzer.)

Although the students completed a yearbook for 1972, it was never published. Fifty years later, the class of 1972 still wonders what happened to it. Although they did not have a yearbook to capture senior year, they certainly had memories. Perhaps this chapter can be considered the 1972 yearbook that was never produced. These students are celebrating a birthday. (Janelle Adamski.)

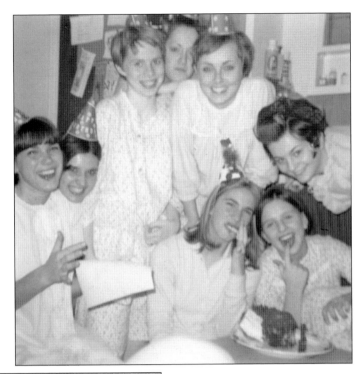

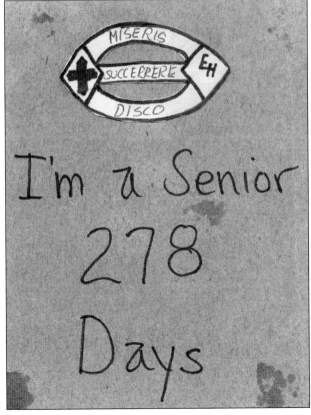

MISERIS
SUCCERRERE EH
DISCO

I'm a Senior
278
Days

Just like that, student nurses became seniors and started counting the days to graduation. The three years went by way too quickly. They made lifelong friends from individuals they did not know three years ago and gained many nursing skills and an abundance of new knowledge. Before the graduation ceremony, many of them took bandage scissors to their student uniforms, as recalled by Cheryl Petersen. (Nancy Miller.)

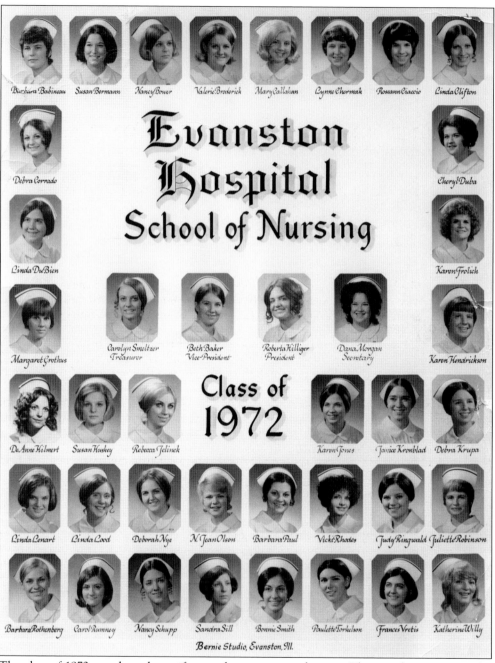

Evanston Hospital School of Nursing

Class of 1972

Barbara Babineau, Susan Bermann, Nancy Bower, Valerie Broderick, Mary Callahan, Lynne Chermak, Roseann Ciaccio, Linda Clifton

Debra Corrado, Cheryl Duba

Linda DuBien, Karen Frolich

Margaret Grothus, Carolyn Smeltzer Treasurer, Beth Baker Vice-President, Roberta Hilliger President, Dana Morgan Secretary, Karen Hendrickson

DeAnne Hilmert, Susan Huskey, Rebecca Jelinek, Karen Jones, Janice Kronblad, Debra Krupa

Linda Lenart, Linda Lood, Deborah Nye, N. Jean Olson, Barbara Paul, Vicki Rhodes, Judy Ringwald, Juliette Robinson

Barbara Rothenberg, Carol Rumney, Nancy Schupp, Sandra Sill, Bonnie Smith, Paulette Torkelson, Frances Vretis, Katherine Willy

Bernie Studio, Evanston, Ill.

The class of 1972 voted on the uniform to be worn at graduation. The cap they wore was the fourth and final cap the school designed. This class actually started out with the third-generation cap, which was discontinued and replaced with one that was easier to clean. The 1972 graduates are pictured here. (Linda Cranford.)

Five

The Impossible Dream
EHSN Graduation 50 Years Later

In 1901, Annie L. Carter and Sarah Elliott became the first two nurses to graduate from the two-year program at Evanston Training School for Nurses. The 1902 class graduated three nurses, and six graduated in 1903. There was no graduating class in 1908, since the curriculum was expanded to three years in 1906.

The first public commencement—for six students—was held on June 17, 1909. The ceremony was held in the women's room at the Evanston YMCA. It included music, flowers, family, friends, and past graduates. Dean Webster presented the diplomas, and the president of the hospitals gave the pins.

The last Patten Hall lawn graduation was held in June 1912. The following graduations were held with Northwestern University graduates at that school, followed by a pinning ceremony at Patten Hall. Amanda Patten, while she was alive, provided the Evanston Hospital nursing pins and placed each pin on the graduate's uniform. When the bachelor's degree program with Northwestern University ceased to exist, the student nursing graduation ceremonies were held in Patten Memorial Hall, the hospital auditorium, or outside.

Prior to a pinning ceremony becoming tradition, students created another tradition of having other students place black bands on each other's caps to signify their length of service as a student. In 1915, this tradition became known as the black band ceremony.

On June 17, 1972, forty students graduated from Evanston Hospital School of Nursing—three were married, two had children, and some were engaged. This was the exact same date, 63 years prior, that the first graduation ceremony for EHSN nursing students was held at the YMCA in Evanston. The 1972 graduation and pinning ceremony were held in the Frank Auditorium of Evanston Hospital.

The following statement is taken from a letter written by Elizabeth Odell, who served as the director of EHSN from 1925 until 1951, and is true for the 1972 class as well as for students prior to 1948: "Evanston Hospital School of Nursing graduates are scattered far and wide. Whether they serve in positions of great responsibility or those of lesser responsibility is not vital. The crucial test is not the importance of their positions, but the quality of their service. The Evanston Hospital School of Nursing has reason to be justly proud of their graduates." Each graduate reached the impossible dream!

TO: Senior Class

FROM: A distinguished resident of 1612 Fargo Ave.

RE: The Festive last gathering

DATED: JUne 8, 1972

Just a reminder that:

   (1) The party is on for Thursday night, June 15th, and full
       attendance is expected

   (2) The time is 8:00 P.M. until the police arrive or sunrise, whichever
       comes first.

   (3) Rare exotic food may be served, the Missouri Giantess may make a
       guest appearance, and those of you not in the best of shape for
       a final blast better start training now.

You know it's time for a wild graduation party if any of the follwing have
ever been true:

(1) Two years ago graduation was your personal version of the impossible dream.

(2) You at one time thought your inferiority complex was bigger and better
    than anybody else's in the School.

(3) Despite problems that were presented to you like a Freudian Smorgasbord,
    you stubbornly survived.

(4) You tended to believe any clump of instructors seen talking were
    talking about you.

(5) You at times had a hard time making your pep pills get a little ahead
    of your tranquilizers.

(6) You almost decided to become a practical nurse by marrying a rich,
    elderly patient.

(7) You think you might miss the lush living quarters upstairs. I know,
    I was upstairs once and tripped over drunk after drunk.

(8) You learned what the school was all about--mainly that it's that big
    building next to the hospital that has at least four sides--on almost
    every issue.

(9) You learned to avoid an emotional crisis while selecting the wrong
    answer.

Dr. Reid James hosted a party for the class of 1972. The invitation listed what the students had accomplished in three years. He was a favorite teacher of most students and was known for making class fun. This image shows the first half of his instructions and invitation. The party was held at his home and was enjoyable. The students requested he be the graduation speaker, but that was not possible. (Katherine Carroll.)

The faculty gave the students a lot of personal attention and personalized all events. This is an invitation sent to Nancy Miller for the cap-striping celebration a year prior to graduation, signed by instructor Marilyn Keyes. Note Keyes's beautiful handwriting. (Nancy Miller.)

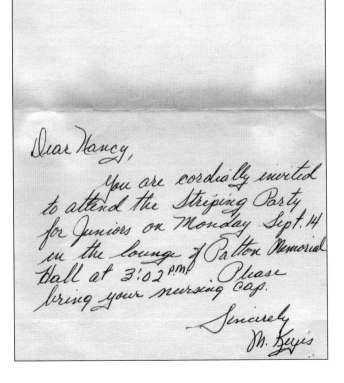

Dear Nancy,

You are cordially invited to attend the Striping Party for Juniors on Monday Sept. 14 in the lounge of Patton Memorial Hall at 3:02 P.M. Please bring your nursing cap.

Sincerely
M. Keyes

The EHSN faculty hosted a breakfast to honor the graduates on the day of their graduation. This was a special but bittersweet time, as students said goodbye to the instructors who taught them how to become a nurse. Chad Friedman and Carolyn Smeltzer are pictured after the breakfast with the windows of Patten Memorial Hall in the background. (Carolyn Smeltzer.)

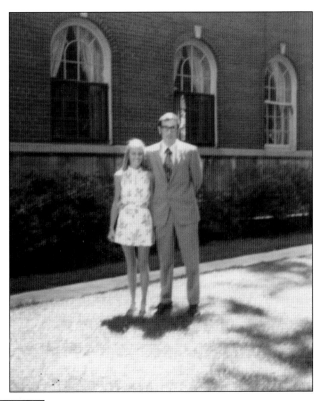

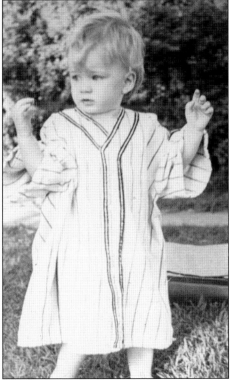

In 1972, EHSN graduation day was especially exciting for Karen Waechter (pictured), whose father, Bill Jones, gave the graduation speech. He used slides to show the "life of a student nurse." As he showed a picture of his daughter, he asked the parents: "Will your little girl grow up and meet Dr. Killdeer, Dr. Joe Gannon, or Ben Casey?" He ended his speech by saying, "With love, Dad." (Karen Waechter.)

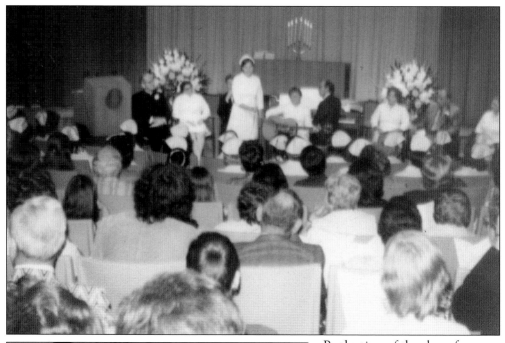

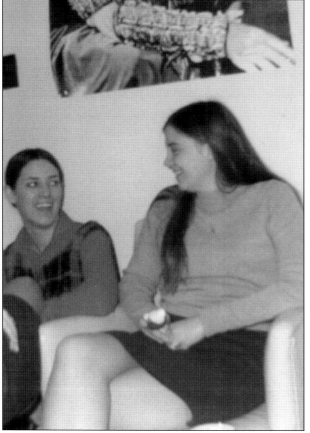

By the time of the class of 1972's golden reunion, three classmates had died. Linda Helgersen DuBien loved children, was mature beyond her age, had loving hands, and was a beautiful singer. She was a nurse practitioner at the University of Chicago Hospital. She tragically died in a car accident at age 28 while Christmas shopping for her three children on Thanksgiving weekend. She is shown singing at graduation. (Linda Cranford.)

After having her second child, Heidi, Linda DuBien opted out of intensive care pediatric nursing because she could not envision her children in an ICU. She and her husband, Larry, moved to Maine and had another child, Joshua. Mathew, her oldest child, died in a snowmobile accident. Today, her fellow class of 1972 students still remember her amazing voice and Mathew. Linda (right) is pictured here with Nancy Miller. (Fran Skafidas.)

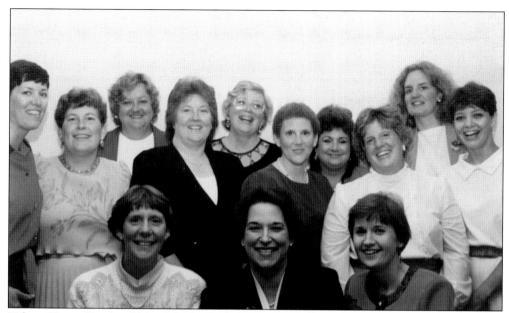

Valerie Karen (Broderick) Metelka had a baby the February before graduation. He was adopted six days later. Years later, Valerie gave birth to Brenda. Valerie died of cervical cancer in 2006. John, her son, had been searching for his birth mother and found his sister through Valerie's obituary—in death, she brought her family together. Valerie is pictured here standing third from left at the school's closing event in 1984. Brenda (Metelka) Ross, owner of Yellow House Bakery, baked the cake for the class's 50th reunion, a skilled she learned from her mother. (Nancy Miller.)

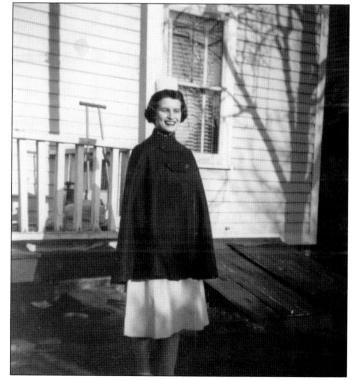

Most of the women in the class of 1972 were born in 1951—the same year that one of their classmates, Juliette La Mar, was enrolled at Grace–New Haven School of Nursing. She was the first and only of seven children to enroll in a higher education program. Even with her good grades, she was forced out of nursing school in her second year after marrying Charles Robinson. (Cameron Vanni.)

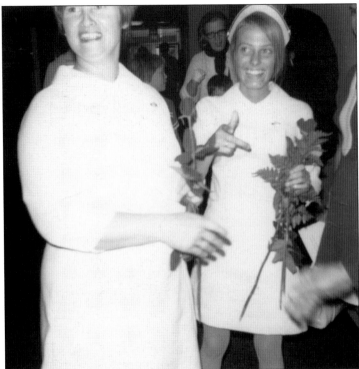

Juliette Robinson pursued her dreams and enrolled at EHSN in 1969. She burned the candle at both ends to make her dream of becoming a nurse come true while raising a family. She was a doctor's wife, a mother of four rambunctious children, had a part-time job, and was a full-time student nurse. Juliette and Carolyn Smeltzer are pictured at EHSN graduation. (Carolyn Smeltzer.)

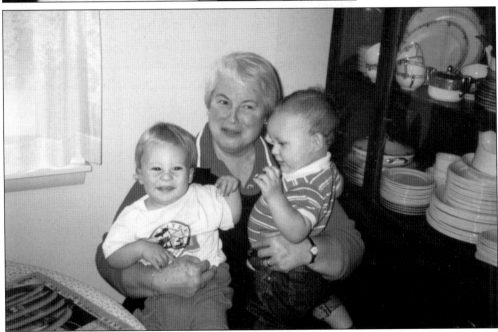

Juliette Robinson studied in the wee hours of the night after finishing her household chores. She had energy, drive, and perseverance, and kept up with her classmates who were 18 years old. Some of her happiest times were spent at Evanston Hospital as a student, caregiver, and supervisor. She died after burying two young sons. Her joy was spending time with her two grandsons, seen here. (Cameron Vanni.)

The 1972 EHSN graduates became administrators, remained staff nurses, practiced for a short time prior to raising a family, and almost all did volunteer work. One student, Roberta Hilliger, followed her love of music, eventually owning a radio station. Pictured from left to right on graduation day are instructor Marilyn Keyes, graduates Barbara McQuillan (who remained at Evanston Hospital for 48 years) and Fran Skafidas (who received a degree from Marycrest College), and instructor Monna Thompson. (Fran Skafidas.)

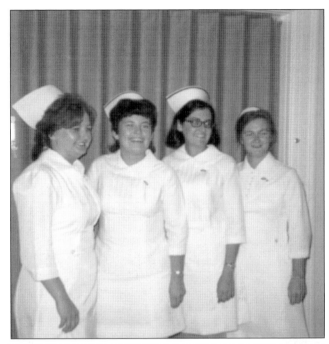

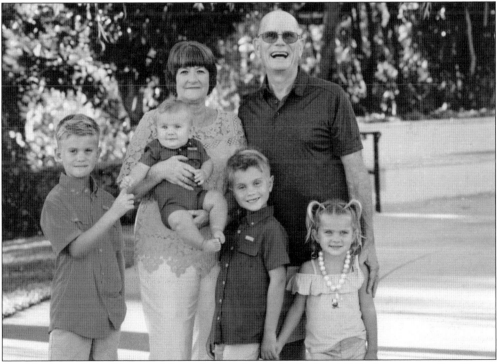

Carol Beebe worked at Evanston Hospital, where she met her husband, Bill, who was attending Garrett Evangelical Theology Seminary. She later worked in Iowa and Florida hospitals. Her nursing career was practiced in the operating room, obstetrical unit, discharge planning department, and oncology unit. She and her husband adopted two children and have four grandchildren. She enjoys traveling, cooking, gardening, and reading, but prefers spending time with her grandchildren. (Carol Beebe.)

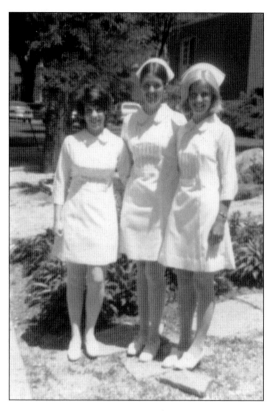

Nancy Miller worked in rehabilitation at Evanston Hospital to fulfill her loan obligations. She became a certified rehabilitation nurse. She and her husband raised and showed bloodhounds. At the birth of her three children was a familiar face—her EHSN classmate Barbara McQuillan. Nancy said, "God blessed me with having Barb being with us on those exciting days" Today, after retirement, she works in a religious education office as a wedding and event coordinator. She is in musical groups and plays bass. Pictured at left from left to right are soon-to-be graduates Roseann Boi, Nancy Miller, and Mary Blaisdell. (Both, Nancy Miller.)

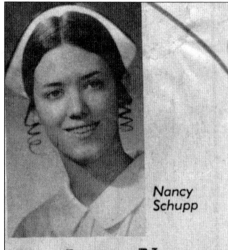

Nancy Schupp

Graduate Nurse

Forty graduating seniors will be awarded diplomas in nursing education from the Evanston Hospital School of Nursing at 1 p.m. Saturday, June 17, in the Frank Auditorium of the hospital.

Among those scheduled to receive her diploma is Nancy J. Schupp, daughter of Mr. and Mrs. Herbert Schupp, of 1418 Second Ave.

Miss Schupp attended Maine Township High School West.

Katherine Carroll is pictured on graduation day. She worked for a private practice of an internist and hematologist. She continued working until 2017. Today, she is in a knitting group and works part-time in the Glenview Park district. (Katherine Carroll.)

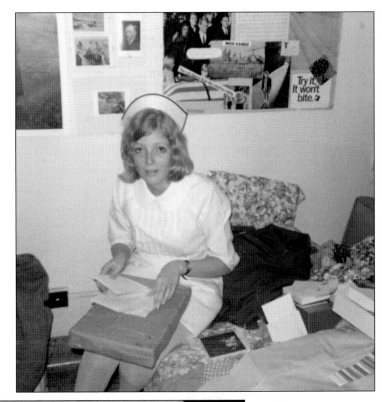

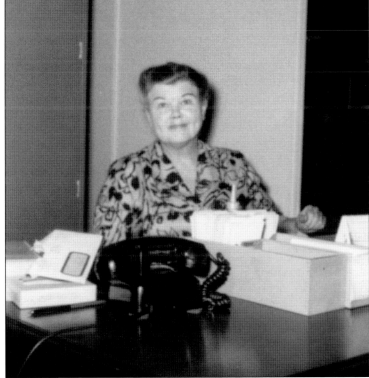

Karen Waechter recalled that she "fell in love with the EHSN library, it was very cozy and homelike." Waechter worked her first 17 years at Northwest Community Hospital and eventually found her passion in hospice nursing. Librarian Louise Monahan, a Michael Reese graduate, is pictured here. (Family of Marjorie Beyers.)

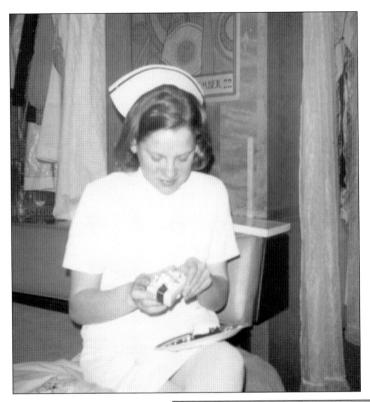

Linda Cranford said, "I had two aunts that were nurses, and I am sure their support and encouragement influenced me to go into nursing. My entire world and life blossomed, and I have never regretted my choice of Evanston Hospital School of Nursing." Cranford is shown opening a gift on graduation day—June 17, 1972. (Carolyn Smeltzer.)

Linda Cranford gave Carolyn Smeltzer a scrapbook as a graduation gift. Inside, a poem read, "Remember? Remember! The day in September. We started the mountain climb. We're finished, yes finished, Three years from '69. We helped each other up, up up." The title of the scrapbook, "To Become a Nurse," was reminiscent of the EHSN brochure "So You Want to Be a Nurse." Both showed up in this book 50 years later. (Carolyn Smeltzer.)

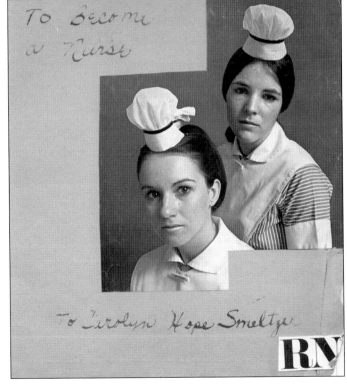

Susan Keenen said, "I have often told people that nursing was my 'founding profession' and that my education and experience provided me with me a 'transferable skill set.'" This is the program for the 1972 graduation. (Katherine Carroll.)

CLASS OF 1972

Candidates for Diploma of Graduate Nurse
◆◆◆◆◆◆◆◆◆◆◆◆◆◆◆◆◆◆◆◆◆◆◆◆

Barbara Ann Babineau
Beth Ann Baker
Susan Iris Bermann
Nancy Ellen Bower
Valerie Karen Broderick
Mary Gerarda Callahan
Lynne Marie Chermak
Roseann Elizabeth Ciaccio
Linda Shaffar Clifton
Debra Corrado
Cheryl Marie Duba
Linda Helgersen DuBien
Karen Lynn Frolich
Margaret E. Grothus
Karen Starr Hendrickson
Roberta Joanne Hilliger
DeAnne Karen Hilmert
Susan Elizabeth Huskey
Rebecca Jane Jelinek
Karen Lynne Jones
Janice Elaine Kronblad
Debra Ruth Krupa
Linda Sue Lenart
Linda Cleveland Lood
Dana Louise Morgan
Deborah Ann Nye
N. Jean Olson
Barbara Leona Paul
Vicki Strotz Rhodes
Judy Jo Ringwald
Juliette LaMar Robinson
Barbara Ann Rothenberg
Carol Ann Rumney
Nancy June Schupp
Sandra Greene Sill
Carolyn Hope Smeltzer
Bonnie Lee Smith
Paulette Marie Torkelson
Frances Marie Vretis
Katherine Anne Willy

The back of the 1972 graduation program includes a poem the class thought best expressed their purpose: "I shall pass through this world but once. If therefore, there be any kindness I can show, or any good thing I can do, let me do it now; let me not defer nor neglect it, for I shall not pass this way again." Pictured is the list of graduates. (Katherine Carroll.)

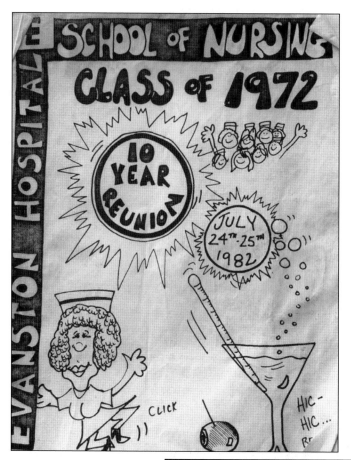

All of the 1972 class members made lifelong friends at school, just like the EHSN brochure said they would. They had their 10th reunion in 1982, and many had no idea that their former school would close just two years later. The graduates all understood the debate about where and how a nurse should be educated. They recalled their faculty encouraging them to go on to college after graduation, which many had done. (Linda Cranford.)

The class of 1972 had a 40-year wait before its next reunion. The 50th reunion was held on Geneva Lake in Wisconsin. They visited George Williams College of Aurora University, which has a nursing program and a patient simulation lab. At one time, this campus was the George Williams YMCA, which pioneered the concept of holistic health. It is interesting to note that the first formal graduation ceremony of EHSN in 1909 was at the Evanston YMCA. Pictured is the class's 10th reunion in 1982. (Linda Cranford.)

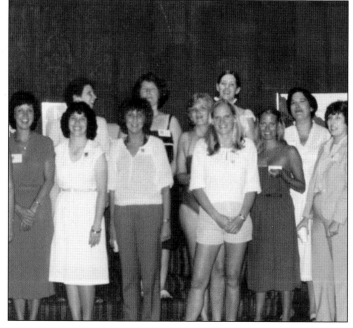

The class of 1972 did as the "So You Want to Be a Nurse" brochure stated, and took opportunities. Some remained staff nurses, while others became nursing administrators, authors, and consultants. Most had families and are now enjoying free time in retirement. All of the 1972 graduates wore their EHSN pins with pride and remembered their fun in the dormitory. (Janelle Adamski.)

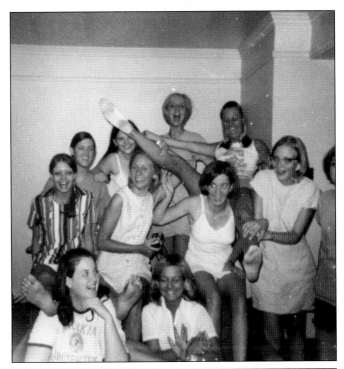

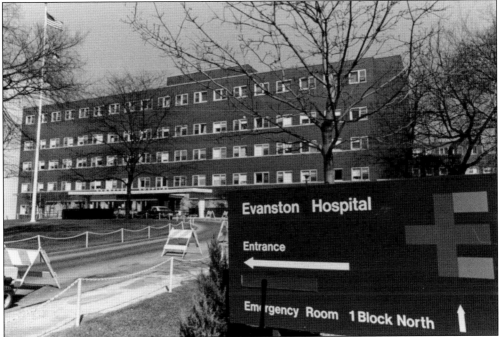

During the 50 years since the 1972 class left EHSN, patient care and the hospital changed. Evanston Hospital, which had 512 beds, is now NorthShore University HealthSystem. The dormitory is now a parking lot, and Evanston Hospital School of Nursing is no longer. The only things that did not change were the EHSN nursing pin and the students' memories. (Archives of Northwestern University.)

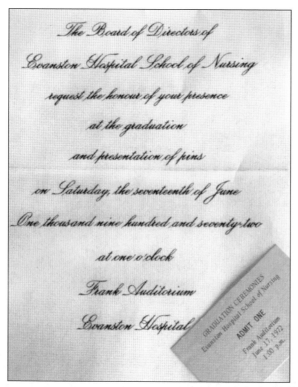

The Board of Directors of

Evanston Hospital School of Nursing

request the honour of your presence

at the graduation

and presentation of pins

on Saturday, the seventeenth of June

One thousand nine hundred and seventy-two

at one o'clock

Frank Auditorium

Evanston Hospital

GRADUATION CEREMONIES
Evanston Hospital School of Nursing
ADMIT ONE
Frank Auditorium
June 17, 1972
1:00 p.m.

With the 1972 graduation invitation came responsibilities for the new nurses. Nursing history was being made without the graduates knowing, as diploma nursing programs were fading, and dormitory life was changing. The song "The Impossible Dream" represented the students' years at EHSN from 1969 to 1972 and how they led their lives of caring as nurses. In the photograph below, Marjorie Beyers (left) is pictured with Rebecca Jelinek-Simon at the Patten Memorial Hall reception after graduation on June 17, 1972. Jelinek-Simon has worked as an ambulatory surgical nurse at Doctors Hospital of Baptist South Florida Health Care for the last 21 years. She has three children and wants to trade her scrubs and surgical gloves for mah-jongg tiles and sunscreen! (Left, Barbara McQuillan and Nancy Miller; below, Rebecca Jelinek-Simon.)

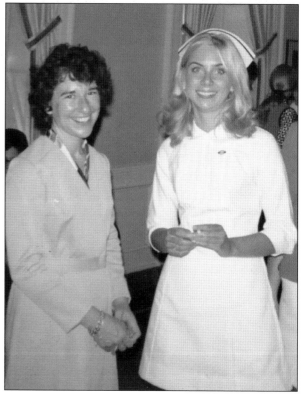

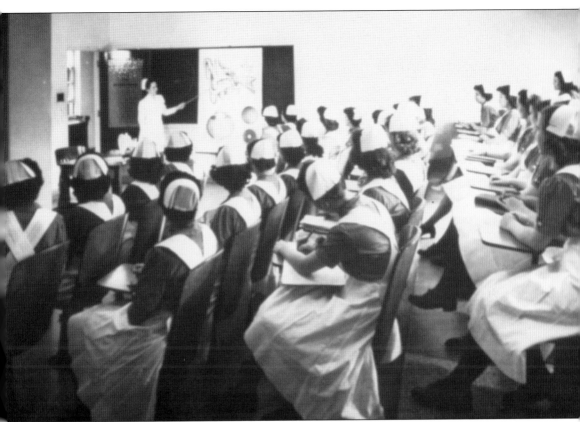

Elizabeth Odell, the longest-serving director of EHSN, wrote these words 76 years ago: "Nursing students are scattered far and wide. Whether they serve in positions involving great responsibilities, or those of lesser responsibilities, is not vital. The crucial test is not the importance of their positions, but rather the quality of service." Authors Carolyn Smeltzer and Barbara McQuillan ask readers to relive and share their own nursing school experiences to keep the history of diploma nursing programs alive.

BIBLIOGRAPHY

"Address to Director of Nursing Service, Massachusetts General Hospital and Associate Director of the American Hospital Association." Nursing Act transcripts, 1964.

Chicago Sun Times, June 14, 1970.

Corry, Sarah. *Notes on Nursing by a Nurse*. New York, NY: D. Appleton-Century, 1944.

Evanston Hospital School of Nursing yearbook, 1970, 1971.

Fairman, Julie and Patricia D'Antonio. "Reimagining Nursing's Place in the History of Clinical Practice." *Journal of the History of Medicine and Allied Sciences*, October 2008.

Gavin, Mary Helt, and Larry Gavin, eds. "15 Stories, 150 Years." *RoundTable*. January 2013.

Hubke, Cindy. *Evanston Hospital School of Nursing Reunion Celebration Book*. November 19, 2020.

Lewenson, Sandra. " 'Nurses' Training May be Shifted': The Story of Bellevue and Hunter College, 1942–1969.' " *Nursing History Review*, volume 21, issue 1, 2013.

Pilot, April 1945, March 1946, April 1961, July 1967.

Putt, Nancy. "Evanston Hospital School of Nursing, 1975–77."

"Review: The Evanston Hospital School of Nursing, 1898–1948." *American Journal of Nursing*, June 1949.

"School of Nursing: A History." *Pilot*, spring 1984.

Schryver, Grace Fay. *A History of the Illinois Training School for Nurses, 1880–1929*. Chicago, IL: Board of Directors of the Illinois Training School for Nurses, 1930.

Sherman, Robert. *All our Past Acclaims our Future: Evanston Hospital, its Standing Today, and What its Future Can Be*. 1940.

Smeltzer, Carolyn Hope, Frances R. Vlasses, and Connie R. Robinson. *Chicago's Nurse Parade*. Charleston, SC: Arcadia Publishing, 2005.

Smeltzer, Carolyn Hope. "The South Side 8: Reflections on Nurses Taken Away Too Soon." www.nurse.com. July 14, 2016.

Smith, Clare Louise. *The Evanston Hospital School of Nursing, 1898-1948*. Chicago, IL: Lakeside Press, 1948.

Thompson, Jenny. "Evanston WWI Veteran Helen Burnett Wood is Honored in America and Scotland." *RoundTable*, November 11, 2021.

Whelan, Jean. "American Nursing: An Introduction to the Past." Penn Nursing, University of Pennsylvania.

ABOUT THE AUTHORS

Carolyn Hope Smeltzer and Barbara Ann McQuillan met in the late summer of 1969 at EHSN. For the next three years, they lived in Patten Memorial Hall together, attended the same classes at EHSN and Northwestern University, learned to care for patients in the same hospital, and celebrated milestones with the same classmates. They said their goodbyes on June 17, 1972, after their graduation ceremony.

Barbara and Carolyn met again at their 10-year reunion. Barbara had remained a nurse at Evanston Hospital, first caring for surgical oncology patients, then changing her specialty to labor and delivery after she visited a classmate in labor. Carolyn had worked on the medical wards at two hospitals, St. Anthony's in Indiana and Billings Hospital of the University of Chicago Medical Center. She had taught nursing at Ravenswood Hospital School of Nursing and was in a nursing leadership role at Foster G. McGaw Hospital, Loyola University of Chicago. Barbara had taken some courses toward a degree, and Carolyn had finished her BS degree at Purdue University and MSN degree at Marcella Niehoff School of Nursing of Loyola University and was enrolled in a doctorate program at Loyola.

During the next four decades, the two had no communication. During those 40 years, Barbara earned the title of diabetes champion for labor and delivery. She met Jim McQuillan on a cruise in 1986, and they married in 1987 and later had two sons. Barbara retired in 2018 after spending 48 years at the same hospital where she trained as a nurse. She now spends her time reading, doing water aerobics, and being with her family, which includes two grandchildren.

Carolyn became a vice president of nursing at two academic medical centers: University of Arizona and University of Chicago. She retired in 2011 as a partner at PricewaterhouseCoopers. Her father stated that she "was on a permanent vacation: golfing, storytelling, serving on healthcare boards, playing bridge, practicing yoga, swimming, and listening to Elvis in her Beetle convertible." Along with coauthors, she has been fortunate to write about three of her passions: nursing, Chicago, and Geneva Lake. Her books include *Ordinary People, Extraordinary Lives: The Stories of Nurses*, *Chicago's Nurse Parade*, *Lake Geneva in Vintage Postcards*, *Geneva Lake*, and *Camps of Geneva Lake*. She married Bob Kelly in 2015, who has always been supportive and understanding of her writing. Carolyn and Bob enjoy spending time with their seven granddaughters.

Barbara and Carolyn started thinking separately about the 50th anniversary of their EHSN graduation. They shared thoughts, located classmates, and collected stories and photographs from their time at EHSN. Both were passionate about EHSN's history and its preservation.

The 50th reunion booklet quickly turned into a history book filled with images and memories. The authors hope this book might encourage all diploma school nursing graduates to tell their unique stories so that future nurses can appreciate this now-extinct type of nursing education. Diploma nursing education holds a proud place in our history. The stories should be told, captured, and not forgotten. This book is a gift to all diploma nurse graduates, especially those from Evanston Hospital School of Nursing.

DISCOVER THOUSANDS OF LOCAL HISTORY BOOKS FEATURING MILLIONS OF VINTAGE IMAGES

Arcadia Publishing, the leading local history publisher in the United States, is committed to making history accessible and meaningful through publishing books that celebrate and preserve the heritage of America's people and places.

Find more books like this at
www.arcadiapublishing.com

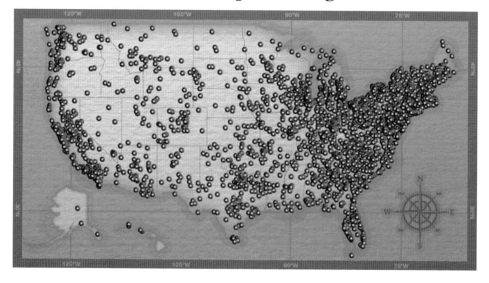

Search for your hometown history, your old stomping grounds, and even your favorite sports team.

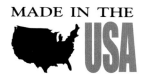